Copyright Notice

Disclaimer

This book is intended as a reference volume only, not as a medical manual. The information given here is designed to help you make informed decisions about your health. It is not intended as a substitute for any treatment that may have been prescribed by your doctor. If you suspect that you have a medical problem, you have to seek medical help.

While thorough attempts have been made to verify the correctness and reliability of the information provided in this publication, the author and publisher do not assume any responsibilities for errors, omissions, or contradictory information contained in this document. The author and publisher are not liable for any losses or damages whatsoever, including but not limited to loss of business, profits, service, clients, information, or any other pecuniary loss.

The information in this book is meant to supplement, not replace, proper exercise training. All forms of exercise pose some inherent risks. All readers are advised to take full responsibility for their safety and know their limits. Be sure that you do not take risks beyond your level of experience, aptitude, training, and fitness. Additionally, the

Table of Contents

About The Author

Before we get started, I would like to thank you for buying this book on patellar tendonitis! The following paragraphs will shed some light on my history, why I decided to write this book, and what you can expect from it.

My name is Martin Koban and I'm a personal trainer from Germany. I've been playing basketball and volleyball for most of my life and after 15 years of enjoying these sports, I eventually developed knee pain. However, it wasn't until my brother tore his meniscus in 2009 during a warm-up for volleyball practice that I finally started to take knee health a lot more seriously.

I figured if such a serious knee injury could happen that easily to him, it could happen to me as well. I therefore began to spend a considerable amount of time reading about knee health in the years that followed.

In 2011, I started www.fix-knee-pain.com to provide a high quality website about knee pain to those looking for answers. At the time of this writing, the website has helped over 800,000 people.

Disappointed with the available books on the topic, I decided to write a book about knee health in 2012. That book, *Total Knee Health: A Radical Approach*, focuses on all the requirements for healthy knees, most of which are completely ignored by other books and by doctors.

The results readers achieved with the techniques described in *Total Knee Health* were exceptional and they are now being used by professional athletes and trainers from around the world. For example, I was invited to share this knowledge with the athletic trainers of the German National Volleyball Team.

I'm tremendously grateful for the opportunity to help so many people. However, I also realize that some questions about patellar tendonitis remained unanswered, which is why I wanted to address this topic with a separate book. This book will help you do two things: it will help you **get back into the game as quickly as possible** and it will help you make sure you **stay healthy.**

What You Can Expect From This Book

In this book, you will learn about the obvious and **hidden causes for patellar tendonitis**. The hidden causes are usually ignored by doctors, but they explain why jumper's knee reappears even after you've been pain-free for some time.

By fixing these hidden causes, you effectively reduce your risk for jumper's knee and you will be able to **prevent it from returning** in the future.

Once we've covered the theory, we'll dive right into the practical application. You will learn a number of exercises that science has proven to be effective for treating jumper's knee, and you'll be given a training program that will help you get your knees healthy again.

Let's get started!

Martin Koban, Berlin August 2013

Chapter 1: Important Fundamentals

This first chapter introduces three important topics that you need to know before you start treating your injury. We will talk about the red flags that clearly show you when you need to go see a doctor, briefly cover what patellar tendonitis is, and go over the symptoms of patellar tendonitis.

Do I Need to See a Doctor?

I received an interesting email from a reader of my email newsletter earlier this year. Apparently, she had suffered a knee injury a few days before and was now hoping that my exercise suggestions could help. I asked her about her pain and it turns out that she had swelling in her knee, could barely walk, and was unable to completely flex or extend the leg. I told her to go see a doctor as soon as possible, to which she merely responded "I guess I knew it all along."

A few days later, I received another mail from her. It turns out she had a torn meniscus!

One great thing about the internet is that you can find information on almost everything. Do you want to know how to breakdance? The internet has you covered. Do you want to diagnose yourself based on some symptoms you have? It's not a problem. What is a problem, however, is that some people, like the lady with the torn meniscus, will try to deal with diseases on their own when they really should seek the help of a medical professional. Don't make that mistake!

Depending on the circumstances under which you first noticed the pain, either you will need to visit a doctor or you can wait and see if the condition improves. Some characteristics of knee pain that will require you to go see a professional:

- You cannot bear weight on the limb

- The knee looks deformed or swollen

- The pain is very severe, keeping you up at night

- The onset of the pain coincided with a fever

- The pain is not improving and is constantly noticeable

- The pain is very sharp

- You cannot fully flex or extend the knee

If you have suffered an acute injury to your knee, regardless of whether it was a contact injury (e.g., someone bumped into your knee) or a non-contact injury (e.g., you landed awkwardly from a jump), you need to have it taken care of by a professional.

If you get hurt during a competitive game, you might be inclined to continue playing out of ego or pride. In that situation, your adrenaline is up and you will not be able to feel most of the pain, meaning the pain will likely get (a lot) worse after the game, especially if you keep playing. Be this as it may, you are probably not a professional athlete. In that case, there's no coaching staff on site, and no medical expert in the locker room. You're also not getting paid millions to wreck your body. The question really is whether you want to **cut your losses and fight another day**, or whether you want to **gamble and risk not being able to play ever again**.

It may sound harsh, but that's the reality of recreational sports. I've known many recreational basketball players who kept playing with pain, never cared for proper recovery, and in the end had to stop playing because their bodies were too beat up to handle it anymore. Ten years down the road, they'll regret this decision, as they can't play with their kids.

In sports, chronic (knee) pain often develops because of a big ego. Make better choices now and you won't have to regret mistakes.

What is Patellar Tendonitis?

The three major bones that make up your knee are the thighbone, the shinbone, and the kneecap. When you extend your knee, your quadriceps, the group of muscles on the front of your thigh, start working. The quads attach to the top-part of your thighbone and your hip on one end and to the kneecap as well as the shinbone on the other end.

If you're contracting your quads, there will be a pull on your kneecap. The purpose of the kneecap is to increase the mechanical advantage of the quadriceps. The kneecap attaches to the shinbone via the patellar tendon and, as you can imagine, the patellar tendon has to be extremely tough to withstand the forces exerted on it through contractions of the quadriceps muscles.

To locate the patellar tendon, sit on a chair with your knee a little bent and relax your legs. Take the same side hand and gently press into the area below your kneecap with your fingers. Everything should be completely relaxed. Now, tense up your leg muscles. Your fingers will feel something tense up below your kneecap. This band of tissue that runs from your kneecap to your shinbone and relaxes when you relax your muscles is the patellar tendon.

Like every other tendon, the patellar tendon can be injured if it's overloaded. This overload can happen during one training session in which your patellar tendon was placed under loads that were cumulatively too high. It can also happen as a result of several training sessions between which you didn't provide your body with enough recovery time. Once overload happens you're dealing with patellar tendonitis, an acute overuse injury to the patellar tendon.

If the patellar tendon is aggravated further, the injury will slowly progress to a more chronic condition usually called tendinosis (N.B.: For the sake of simplicity, I mostly use the term "patellar tendonitis" or "Jumper's Knee" in this book. Another term you will find in the literature is tendinopathy, which is the umbrella term for injuries to tendons and includes both the acute and the chronic condition).

In other words, patellar tendonitis is the result of your patellar tendon not being strong enough for the demands of your sport. It's the equivalent of failing a test (i.e., playing your sport as a test on your body) because you didn't study enough (i.e., your patellar tendon wasn't strong enough for the test).

If you retake the test without having studied more (i.e., strengthened your patellar tendon), you're going to fail again. Fail a test enough times and you eventually fail school (i.e., the damage to the tendon becomes permanent).

Unfortunately, many athletes are so enthusiastic about their sport that they don't allow their body to heal the damage properly before they jump back into the game. With repeated tissue damage, cellular degradation sets in. The body is unable to repair the injured tissue and a painful chronic condition is created that will take at least three months to heal (Wilson, Best 2005; Khan et al. 1998, p. 348).

If you continue playing, your patellar tendon will continue breaking down, making it even weaker. This increases the risk of a patellar tendon tear, and increases the time ultimately needed to heal it, once you finally decide to take action. To get healthy, you need to stop participating in your sport, go through a progressive strengthening regimen for your patellar tendon, and fix biomechanical mistakes that contributed to the tendon becoming overloaded. The following chapters will help you do just that and give you the information you need to **stay pain-free for life.**

The Symptoms of Jumper's Knee

The symptoms for patellar tendonitis are pain on the side of, in front of, below, or even behind the kneecap. However, most commonly the pain will reside below the kneecap, where the patellar tendon attaches to the kneecap. Additionally, you may feel tenderness below the kneecap and in the area of the bony protrusion right below. Sometimes the patellar tendon is swollen.

If you have pain in the back of your knee or on the side of your knee, you are likely dealing with a different knee injury. Consult an experienced medical professional to make sure you're not treating the wrong injury.

In patellar tendonitis, pain usually gets worse with activities where energy is stored in the tendon and released more explosively. Such activities include running, climbing stairs, walking downhill and – of course – jumping. Another activity that can worsen the pain is squatting.

Depending on which stage of the injury you are in, the severity of the symptoms will be different. In the early stages, you only feel discomfort after activities that stress your knees. Once the injury has progressed, you may feel pain during the day, which worsens after activities that stress your knees. Additionally, there may be morning stiffness and swelling of the patellar tendon.

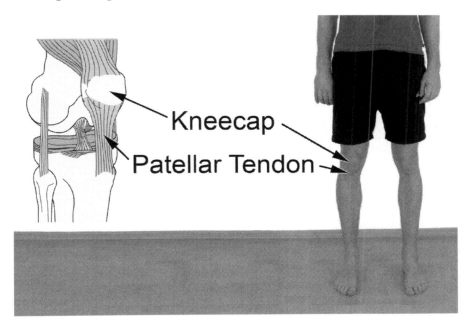

Kneecap

Patellar Tendon

Chapter 2: Tendon Injuries Explained

In this chapter, we will first investigate how tendons are injured and then use that knowledge to understand how your patellar tendon can break down. Next, we will talk about how much treatment time you can expect.

How Tendon Injuries Occur

Tendons connect muscles to joints, thereby allowing us to move our skeleton through muscle contractions. Tendons consist of collagen fibers, which can withstand impressive forces because of their high tensile strength (Kannus 2000). Tensile strength is the maximum force a material can be subjected to before breaking. Additionally, collagen fibers are like small rubber bands since they can store elastic energy.

Like most tissues of the human body, tendons grow stronger to meet the demands we place upon them (Reeves et al. 2003). The problem is that tendons and ligaments are slow to adapt. Muscle function adapts much faster to a training stimulus, which allows us to exert forces on our tendons that can exceed their capacity for load (Kubo et al. 2010).

If we progress slowly in our training, giving our tendons enough time to "catch up" with our improved muscle function and increased force output, we can prevent tendon injuries from happening. However, the competitive nature of sports and the fact that many of us simply enjoy movement makes curbing the enthusiasm for fast progress and a high level of activity difficult.

A contributing problem is that once you feel pain, tendon damage is already substantial (Khan et al. 1998, p. 351). In other words, just because you're not in pain, doesn't mean your patellar tendon has not degenerated to some degree. Hence, pain is only a delayed indicator of whether an activity is safe to perform or not. This is also demonstrated by the fact that Achilles tendon ruptures often occur without any warning; the tendon becomes weak due to degeneration without being painful.

The Pathology Continuum of Tendon Injuries

The research on patellar tendonitis predominantly distinguishes between injury stages based on when you feel the pain, or whether the pain is limiting your performance (Rutland et al. 2010). However, these models leave several important questions unanswered, particularly when it comes to the best way of treating patellar tendonitis, which is why I prefer a newer model.

At the time of writing, a recently proposed tendinopathy continuum model by Dr. Jill Cook (Monash University, Australia) seems best suited to explain the changes inside a tendon caused by overload. This model distinguishes between four stages of tendon health based on the actual cellular changes within the tendon: a normal tendon, reactive tendinopathy, tendon dysrepair, and degenerative tendinopathy (Cook, Purdam 2009, p. 409).

Please note that not all parts of the tendon progress through these stages at the same speed. Parts of the tendon may still be healthy while other parts have already advanced into stages of injury.

Let's look at the three injury stages in a bit more detail and then talk about how you can use these findings to determine the best treatment option for your particular case of patellar tendonitis.

Reactive Tendinopathy: The Minimally Injured Tendon

A tendon progresses from the normal stage to reactive tendinopathy when it has been exposed to excessive loads without allowing adequate time for recovery. This stage is called reactive tendinopathy because the cells of the tendon have become reactive in an effort to repair damage done to the tendon.

Imagine you usually play your sport, say volleyball or basketball, twice per week for one hour. You knees are completely fine with that load, as the training schedule allows adequate time for recovery and the training volume is not excessive.

However, over the weekend your team participates in a tournament that lasts from 10 AM in the morning to 6 PM in the evening. You may end up playing four or more hours during the tournament and, while your muscles have enough time to recover between games, your patellar tendon can't keep up. At the end of the tournament, you've placed excessive cumulative load on it and forced your tendon into the reactive tendinopathy stage.

In reactive tendinopathy your tendon thickens somewhat. This is the body's stop-gap solution to deal with the excessive stress until a more permanent adaptation can take place. Tendon cells change their shape to increase protein production, and more water is bound in the tendon. The integrity of the collagen fibers in your tendon doesn't change and the tendon can return to the normal stage if the load is reduced appropriately (Cook, Purdam 2009, p. 410).

Since the collagen alignment doesn't change, the tensile strength of the tendon doesn't decrease. Therefore, you can keep playing without a drop in performance, although your tendon might be a bit achy after the game.

By the way, a blow to your tendon can also lead to reactive tendinopathy because such trauma results in the same tendon response (Garau et al. 2008, p. 1616). Additionally, if you've taken considerable time off from training and return to your previous training volume too quickly, you can end up with reactive tendinopathy. This is because your tendon has grown weaker during the time off from training since no loads were placed on it (Yamamoto et al. 1999).

Tendon Dysrepair: You've Abused the Tendon More Than Once

The tendon progresses from reactive tendinopathy to tendon dysrepair, the second injury stage, if the load wasn't reduced adequately or if not enough time for recovery was allowed after the initial overload occurred.

Returning to the example of the weekend tournament, imagine you wake up on Monday and one of your patellar tendons is a bit achy. Your usual training schedule calls for sessions on Monday and Thursday, and you don't want to miss either of them. You decide to ignore your achy knee and play regardless. Maybe you even take some medication to deal with the pain.

Unfortunately, your tendon hasn't recovered from the weekend tournament yet, and the continued jumping and running will damage it further. You stay on your training schedule for weeks even though your tendon is still achy.

Inside the tendon, the number of tendon cells has increased, just like the protein production. The collagen has started to become disorganized and, as result, tensile strength has decreased. At this stage, the tendon is more susceptible to overload and the level of activity that will do damage to it is lower than in a healthy tendon (Khan et al. 1998, p. 348). In other words, the level of activity that wasn't a problem before the tournament now places too much stress on your tendon.

Depending on how deep you've progressed into this stage, your tendon can still be healed if you stick to an intelligent exercise regime and stop all activities that overload your tendon. Recovery will take longer and has to be approached carefully however.

Degenerative Tendinopathy: Your Tendon Slowly Dies

If you keep overstressing your tendon, the injury will progress into the degenerative stage. Cells within the tendon have already died and continue to die. Collagen fiber alignment is chaotic. The tendon's ability to heal is severely compromised and the tensile strength has dropped considerably. Overload may now lead to tendon rupture.

You will reach this stage if you continue to play through pain. For example, say you keep playing on your schedule in spite of the achiness in your knee. A new tournament comes up and even though you have doubts about whether you should participate, you don't want to leave your team hanging. Let's face it: they don't stand much of a chance without you. After the tournament, the pain got worse, but you, being as tough as nails, still stay on your weekly training schedule.

This cycle continues for months and the pain gets a little worse with each passing week. A few months and another couple of tournaments down the road, your knee hurts all the time. Normal daily activities like sitting or walking down stairs cause pain. You finally take time off from training.

The following figure illustrates the progression through the individual stages of health. I adapted it from Dr. Cook's research paper on the tendinopathy continuum (Cook, Purdam 2009, p. 410).

Stronger Tendon

Normal Tendon

Reactive Tendinopathy

Tendon Dysrepair

Degenerative Tendinopathy

Appropriate Load

Stage-Based Treatment of Tendinopathy

It is difficult to determine which exact stage of tendinopathy an injured tendon is in, especially since parts of the tendon can be in different stages and the only evident symptom is pain, which can occur in all stages. For this reason, Cook suggests dividing the injury continuum into reactive tendinopathy/early tendon dysrepair and late tendon dysrepair/degenerative tendinopathy (Cook, Purdam 2009, p. 415).

This simplification makes sense since early in the injury stage parts of the tendon will be in the reactive phase, whereas other parts might already be in early tendon dysrepair. Once the injury progresses and most parts of the tendon are in dysrepair, some parts will already be in degenerative tendinopathy.

Let's look at the best treatments for each stage and then talk about how much treatment time you can expect.

Treatment for Reactive Tendinopathy and Early Tendon Dysrepair

In this stage, the tendon is still able to heal itself. There is no need for exercises like eccentric squats that specifically target the tendon. All you need to do is to reduce the load to appropriate levels and to allow adequate time for recovery. This will lead to your tendon cells becoming less reactive and pain will be reduced as well (Cook, Purdam 2009, p. 413).

One way you can determine whether you're in this phase (other than diagnostic imaging) is by remembering the first time you had pain or discomfort in your tendon. If it was no more than a few weeks in the past, you very likely are in this stage.

Going back to the earlier example, you could take a week off from training and only do technique drills for the two weeks that follow. Slowly return to your previous schedule once your pain is gone. You need to monitor your condition. Whenever an exercise increases your pain, meaning you have more pain a few hours after the exercise than you had before, you need to modify that exercise. To do that, train for a shorter amount of time or do less intense exercises.

For example, the first time you train again after your week off you should take it easy and reduce the training time during which you stress your knees, let's say to 20 minutes. For the remaining time of your training, you can do technique drills that don't overload your knees. Increase the length of the part of the training during which you stress your knees by 10% each week. Hence, you'd do 22 minutes in the second week, 32 minutes in the fifth week, and so on. After 12 weeks, you're back at 60 minutes of intense movement per session.

When you're in this stage, allow at least two or three days for recovery between sessions that stress your knees. If you want to practice your sport more often, limit your training to practicing the technique without placing load on your knees.

In addition to modifying your training load, you need to fix all factors that contribute to patellar tendonitis. These factors determine how much load your patellar tendon has to handle during athletic movements, and you can considerably reduce your risk of patellar tendon overload by addressing them. You will learn more about these critically important factors in the following chapters.

For many athletes, fixing these factors alone can be the difference between staying healthy and developing jumper's knee.

Treatment for Late Tendon Dysrepair and Degenerative Tendinopathy

In this stage, the tendon is no longer fully able to heal itself. You need to implement exercises that specifically target the tendon and trigger collagen formation (Cook, Purdam 2009, p. 413). In addition, you need refrain from all unnecessary exercises that cause increased pain in your tendon.

You're in this stage if you kept playing at a high intensity level for months after the initial onset of discomfort in your knee. The exact amount of time it takes depends on the weekly exposure to overload. An athlete that trains through pain four times per week will obviously progress faster than someone who "only" trains through pain twice per week.

Another indicator that you're in this stage is if you've had tendon pain several times in the past. Back then, the pain resolved but then reoccurred once you resumed your training (Cook, Purdam 2009, p. 411). This is because your tendon is already weakened and its tensile strength has decreased because the collagen alignment is disorganized. The weakened tendon cannot handle normal training loads, which is why training leads to a return of pain.

In this stage, the tendon will not heal on its own. You will need to do certain exercises to restart the healing process. We will talk about these exercises in a later chapter.

Please don't forget that tendon degeneration can also occur without pain. For example, one study found that two-thirds of tendons that were degenerated enough to rupture were pain-free (Kannus, Józsa 1991). However, since you're likely reading this book because you are in pain, you can use the onset of pain or discomfort to tell how far you've progressed in the tendinopathy continuum.

Is There Inflammation?

Initially, tendonitis was believed to be an inflammatory response of the body to the overload of the tendon, which is why the disease carries the suffix "–itis" in its name. However, as scientific methods progressed, tendonitis was found to be mostly void of inflammation.

Dr. Jill Cook points out that tendonitis is an activated cell response, not an inflammatory response. In the initial phase of the disease, reactive tendinopathy, taking anti-inflammatories such as NSAIDs and corticosteroids can be beneficial. However, this isn't because of their anti-inflammatory properties per se, but because they inhibit the cell response of the reactive cells to a certain degree. Since in the advanced stages of tendinopathy you want your tendon cells to be reactive, these treatment options are not recommended.

Cook concludes her paper on the tendinopathy continuum by pointing out that there may be "some form of inflammation" in tendinopathy, but the finer details are unclear (Cook, Purdam 2009, p. 415). So far, no ultimate consensus has been reached about the exact role of inflammation in tendinopathy (Rees et al. 2013).

How Much Treatment Time Will it Take?

Giving a time estimate on how long treatment will take is difficult (Cook, Purdam 2009, p. 415), but in research studies pain noticeably improved in the first 3 to 4 weeks and most studies ran for 12 weeks (Rutland et al. 2010).

Treatment time depends on how far you've progressed in the injury stages. Athletes in the reactive tendinopathy/early dysrepair stage will likely be back on the court within 4 to 8 weeks. In contrast, athletes who have let their injury progress into the advanced stages are looking at three or more months of treatment.

Treatment of patellar tendonitis is a slow process. You're moving upward in the tendinopathy continuum, slowly allowing all parts of your tendon to recover from the dysrepair stage, to the reactive tendinopathy stage, until they are finally at the normal stage again. How much time this takes strongly depends on how severely your tendons are injured.

Additionally, even once your tendons are in the normal stage of the injury continuum, they might still be too weak for your particular sport. If your tendons are pain-free, but pain returns once you take up your sport again, you know that you need to strengthen them further. You can do this with the tendon strengthening exercises in this book, or you can scale your sporting activity down to a level at which your pain does not return.

A later chapter will explain how you can keep playing your sport in spite of jumper's knee.

In summary, if you just want to get rid of the pain, four to eight weeks of strengthening your knees is likely all you need. If you want your knees to be strong enough to handle a 40-inch vertical leap, you might have to continue the tendon strengthening for much longer.

Lastly, the question about treatment time always implies a certain sense of urgency. I understand that sense of urgency, as I myself have played basketball competitively, albeit in a minor league.

Sports are fun and you don't want to let your teammates hanging. In the end, however, it boils down to one simple question: are you a recreational athlete or a pro-athlete? That is, do you compete just for fun or are you being paid to compete?

At first glance, you might not agree with the importance of that distinction, after all, pros play the very same game as recreational athletes, so what's the difference?

The difference is that a pro-athlete puts his body at risk because he is being paid to entertain people. The harsh reality is that professional athletes are the modern day gladiators. They make a living because we enjoy watching them do what they do. The fewer people enjoy watching a particular sport, the less money is in it. Sure, many pro-athletes love their sport, but let's be honest here, how many of them would be spending 8 hours a day training if they weren't being paid to do so?

Since pro-athletes are a significant financial investment for their particular teams, there's a need to provide the athlete with the best care possible. They have a highly qualified athletic staff on hand and they have dialed their nutrition in to support their health as best as possible.

The recreational athlete, on the other hand, plays sports for fun and maybe because he wants to stay in shape. Staying in shape requires you to stay healthy and staying healthy requires you not to be injured because of dumb mistakes. These mistakes can be an extra set in the weight room after you felt like you should stop, or an extra 30 minutes on the court after you felt that you were already too tired to compete.

Risking injury defeats the purpose of recreational sports, because an injury isn't fun and it's not good for your health either.

Since you're reading this book, you're probably better than most of your competition anyway, simply because you put time into educating yourself to become a better athlete. There's no need to risk your potential by being sucked into some ego-driven competition, or by trying to recover too quickly from an injury.

Play it safe today and people may call you lame, but a few months down the road, you'll kick their asses. Remember that only slow and steady wins the game when it comes to recovering from patellar tendonitis.

Let's now talk about the causes for jumper's knee.

Chapter 3: Obvious and Hidden Causes of Jumper's Knee

In this chapter, we will investigate the obvious and hidden causes for jumper's knee. If you've done some prior reading about jumper's knee, on the internet or in other books, you will know that the commonly given advice is to rest. This is useful advice, but it is missing an explanation of the biomechanical factors that contribute to jumper's knee.

If you don't fix these biomechanical problems, your patellar tendonitis will return eventually. We will look at these critical factors in the second part of this chapter. For now, let's talk about primary cause for jumper's knee.

Understanding the Primary Cause of Jumper's Knee

Patellar tendonitis is very common in sports that require a lot of jumping, such as volleyball and basketball (Lian et al. 2005), but it also occurs in soccer players (Hägglund et al. 2011), dancers, weightlifters, and other sports in which a lot of kicking, sprinting, and running is done (Rutland et al. 2010).

In essence, all sports that require work from the knee extensors will place a high load on your patellar tendon (Frohm et al. 2007). Let's take a closer look at jumping and the two main sports associated with it, volleyball and basketball.

The rapid acceleration and deceleration that takes place when you're jumping and landing exerts a force of around 6- to 7-times bodyweight on the patellar tendon, although other activities such as running and weightlifting also place a lot of load on it (Rutland et al. 2010). Under ideal circumstances, the tendon would be able to adapt during your rest period, but if you repeatedly place too much stress on your tendon without giving it enough time to recover, it will start to break down.

For example, a study on elite female basketball players with patellar tendinopathy found that players with patellar tendonitis in one or both knees trained one to three hours more per week on average when compared to their healthy teammates (Gaida et al. 2004).

Another study, performed on amateur volleyball players in Norway, found that players with patellar tendonitis performed more weight training per week than their healthy teammates (Tiemessen et al. 2009).

The Norwegian study also revealed that athletes with jumper's knee had a higher vertical leap and stronger legs, likely because they put in more work in the weight room (Lian et al. 2003), which ties in nicely with what you've learned in the subchapter on how tendon injuries occur: the muscles get too strong and your tendons cannot keep up. As a result, your muscles are able to make your tendons work harder than they can, making it easy for you to overload them with too much volume too quickly.

The amount of training volume it takes to do damage to the tendon is highly individual. It depends on the athlete's ability to recover, nutrition, their movement quality, and a host of other factors. If you look at the subjects from the two previously mentioned studies again, you will find some healthy athletes that train more hours per week than their injured colleagues do. Hence, although a higher volume of weekly training is a risk factor for developing patellar tendonitis, there's no such thing as a magic number of training hours you shouldn't exceed if you want to stay healthy.

In summary, the primary cause for patellar tendonitis is overload of the patellar tendon. Training too often without giving the tendon enough time to recover will eventually lead to jumper's knee. This overload occurs silently because you will only feel pain once damage has already been done to the tendon (Khan et al. 1998, p. 351; Huisman et al. 2013).

In other words, even if your knees are fine, your patellar tendon could already be damaged. Additionally, if you've suffered from patellar tendonitis and have progressed in the rehab process to a point at which you're pain-free, you'd still be well advised to continue your tendon strengthening for another couple of weeks because being pain-free doesn't mean your tendon is 100% healthy again.

9 Hidden Causes for Patellar Tendonitis

The patellar tendon always has to handle at least some load when you're moving. However, there are certain factors that influence how much load your tendons have to deal with. Addressing these factors can help you lower your risk for jumper's knee in the future and can be the decisive difference for the success of your treatment.

Each of these factors will be addressed with the exercises provided in a later chapter. For now, let's just look at the theory behind these factors.

1) Low Ankle Dorsiflexion

You dorsiflex your ankle when you pull your foot up towards your knee. The opposite movement, plantarflexion, occurs when you point your foot away from your knee. Dorsiflexion happens at the ankle when you bring your knee out over your toes, whereas plantarflexion would be to stand on the balls of your feet.

Decreased ankle dorsiflexion range of motion has been linked with an increased risk for patellar tendonitis in basketball players (Backman, Danielson 2011) and volleyball players (Malliaras et al. 2006). Hence, improving ankle mobility, particularly dorsiflexion, has to be part of a treatment program for patellar tendonitis.

2) Tight Calves

The gastrocnemius muscle in the calves stretches across the knee on the back of your leg. If your gastrocnemius is tight, your knee will always have to work against additional resistance when extending. Massaging and stretching the gastrocnemius is therefore important for keeping undue load off your patellar tendon.

If your calf tightness reoccurs in spite of massage, ankle mobility drills, and stretching, there might be an underlying muscular dysfunction. This dysfunction is causing the tightness of your calves and without fixing this underlying cause, you won't be able to relieve the tightness of your calves. The same holds true for tightness in other muscle groups like your quads or hamstrings.

These kinds of dysfunctions are hard to identify by yourself, which is why you should seek the help of a qualified medical professional such as a Neurokinetic Therapy practitioner (neurokinetictherapy.com).

3) Tight Quadriceps Muscles

Another risk factor for developing patellar tendonitis is tight quadriceps muscles (Mann et al. 2013). Relieving excess tension in your quads will reduce some of the permanent tension your patellar tendon has to handle.

Additionally, tight quads will neurologically inhibit and weaken your hamstring and gluteal muscles. Fixing this problem will allow you to redistribute load to the back of your leg whenever you're moving, which further reduces the load on the patellar tendon.

4) Tight Hamstrings

Just like the gastrocnemius in the calves, the hamstring muscle group crosses the knee on the back of your leg. If your hamstrings are tight, you will always have to work against additional resistance when extending your leg, which puts undue load on your patellar tendon.

Additionally, tight hamstrings will make it difficult for you to properly hinge at the hip, which is the crucial part of proper jumping mechanics. Lack of hip flexion during jumping movements has been indicated as a risk factor for developing patellar tendonitis (Mann et al. 2013). We will talk about the hip hinge in more detail in a later chapter.

Lastly, hamstring tightness can be caused by weak gluteal muscles. Since the hamstrings and glutes are both responsible for creating hip extension, weak gluteals will lead to an increased load on your hamstrings, which is why they become overworked and get tight. For this reason, you should wait to stretch your hamstrings until you've improved gluteal strength and hip mobility.

5) Weak Gluteal Muscles

Research has shown that a weakness in hip abduction and hip external rotation strength is a risk factor for knee pain (Ireland et al. 2003;

Powers 2010). Weak gluteal muscles can contribute to patellar tendon overload in a number of ways. For example, your gluteal muscles control the movement of your thigh when you're running, jumping, or landing from a jump. Therefore, weak gluteals mean you have less control over your thigh movement, increasing the possibility that your knees will cave in towards the midline of your body when running or jumping (internal rotation and adduction).

Having your knees cave inward will cause the patellar tendon to pull off-axis, thereby contributing to tendon overload.

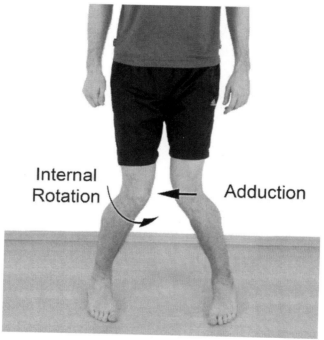

Picture: both thighs are internally rotated and adducted (the arrows illustrate the respective movements)

Additionally, if you have weak gluteals, your body predominantly relies on your quadriceps muscle if you want to run or jump. Since the muscles on the back of your hips and legs are weak, the body compensates by placing more load on those muscle on the front of your thigh and hip, as these are strong. This alone can cause enough additional stress on your knees for you to develop patellar tendonitis.

To remedy this situation, you need to balance the ratio between knee-dominant (exercises that stress the quads more than the glutes and hamstrings) and hip-dominant training (exercises that stress the glutes and hamstrings more than the quads).

6) Low Hip Mobility

If your hip is stiff, you will have difficulty controlling the movement of your thighs when you run, jump, and squat. This is because the stiff muscles oppose those that are trying to create the required movement. With low hip mobility, your risk of ending up with your knees caved in increases and you'll place more load on your knees, particularly your patellar tendon and ACL. Additionally, a stiff hip might give you lower back pain, as the body makes up for the range of motion you're missing at the hip by increase range of motion at the neighboring joints (i.e., the knee and the lower back).

A stiff hip will also limit your success of strengthening your gluteal muscles. This is because the ability to create force through a certain muscle is decreased neurologically if that particular muscle's antagonist (i.e., the muscle that creates the opposing movement) is tight. For this reason, you should always train hip mobility in concert with gluteal strengthening exercises.

As you can see, factors four, five and six are closely related. You need to address all of them if you want to achieve the best results for each individual factor.

7) Wrong Foot Alignment

Another common mistake that many people make is moving with their feet turned out. Turning your feet out during athletic movements will make it easier for your ankle to collapse, which then puts you into an unstable position and places more load on the joints further up (Starrett, Cordoza 2013, pp. 92f). Not only are you limiting your athletic potential by moving with your feet turned out, but you're also increasing your risk of injury.

Please note that you don't have point your feet absolutely straight ahead. You can turn them out to around 5 to 12 degrees and still minimize the negative effects mentioned in the previous paragraph (Starrett, Cordoza 2013, p. 86). However, during practice, I try to maintain the best alignment possible. My reasoning is that once there's some metabolic demand or during the stress of the game, my movement is going to deviate from the ideal anyway and I'd rather have a buffer if that happens. If I practice with my feet pointing almost straight ahead and my feet turn out a little more during the game, I'm still in the safe range.

One common reason why people move this way is because they have limited ankle dorsiflexion range of motion (remember, factor #1) and their body compensates by turning their feet out. This means that you have to work on ankle dorsiflexion to allow for good foot alignment.

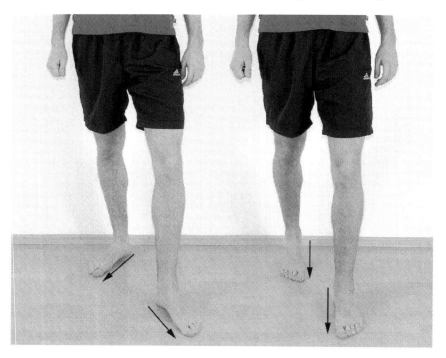

The previous picture illustrates improper foot alignment (left) and proper foot alignment (right). Pay attention to other people's feet the next time you go to the mall and you'll be amazed how many people walk like ducks. Don't be one of them.

8) Wrong Jumping Technique

The technique you use for jumping determines how the load will be distributed throughout your body. If your hamstrings and glutes are weak, you're likely to jump by using the muscles on the front of your thigh (quads). This is because your body compensates for the weak muscles by placing more load on the muscles that are strong, leading to the weight being shifted forward.

This quad-dominant jumping technique slowly overloads your patellar tendon and thereby contributes to patellar tendonitis. This factor can have a big enough impact to cause patellar tendonitis on its own, so you should definitely take it seriously. Conversely, many athletes will find relief from jumper's knee just by fixing this one factor.

Aside from this biomechanical explanation, studies have also identified a correlation between knee angle when landing and patellar tendonitis (Lavagnino et al. 2008). The conclusion is that more of the momentum is absorbed by the hamstrings and glutes if you're hinging at the hip, whereas more of the momentum is absorbed by the quads if you don't hinge enough at the hip. Placing more load on the quadriceps muscles also stresses the patellar tendon more.

Below are pictures illustrating improper jumping technique (knees travel forward or cave inwards) and proper jumping technique (you hinge at the hip, your shins stay vertical, knees don't move forward much and stay above the toes). Please note: you can also hinge much further, until your torso is almost parallel to the ground, depending on how high you jump.

We will talk more about jumping technique in the later chapters.

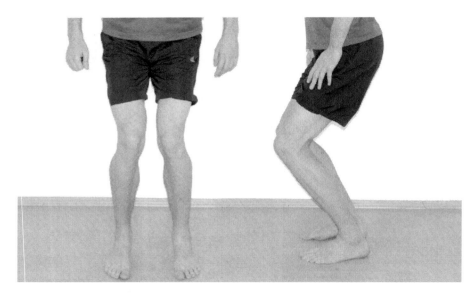

Picture: On the left, knees are collapsed inward. On the right, knees travel too far forward. Both are common jumping technique mistakes.

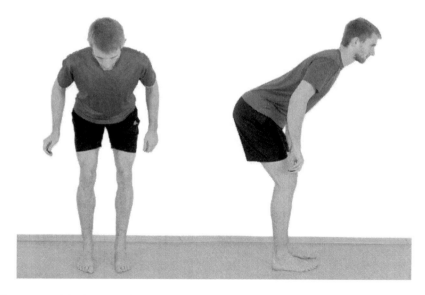

Picture: This image shows a much better jumping technique with the knees aligned above the toes and hinging at the hip.

9) Overtraining / Too Much Too Soon

To understand overtraining, you have to understand how stimuli cause your body to adapt. Whenever we use our body to perform a task, your body's systems react by adapting to the task. If you lift weights, your muscles will grow and you will get stronger. However, the muscles don't grow during training, but after. Lifting weights actually "breaks" muscle down.

Your body wants to make your life easier, so it strengthens the involved tissues once the stimulus has stopped. Muscles grow, tendons get stronger, and bones become denser. The amount of time the body requires to achieve this adaptation depends on a number of factors like training intensity and your individual ability to recover. We all recover at a different pace due to different stress levels, nutrition, and genetic make-up, among other factors.

All subsystems of the body adapt at a different pace. Our nervous system adapts the quickest, followed by our muscles. Tendons and bones take much longer to adapt to training stimuli.

Overtraining occurs when we repeatedly exceed our body's ability to recover from training. We exceed our ability to recover if we train again before the last adaptation was complete.

Applied to patellar tendonitis, you'd be overtraining when you place high loads on your patellar tendons without allowing them proper time for recovery. Inside your tendons, collagen synthesis only reaches a positive net value 36 hours after an intense exercise session (Magnusson et al. 2010). That means if you stress your patellar tendon a lot on consecutive days, you're not giving it enough time to recover fully. If you were to continue this process, the tendons would eventually dip into the reactive tendinopathy stage.

Too much too soon, on the other hand, occurs when you subject your patellar tendons to too much stress during one training session. For example, imagine you're used to practicing your sport for 60 minutes and on one day, you do 120 minutes instead. As you become fatigued, your movement quality decreases and you'll place more load on the patellar tendon.

A similar overload occurs when you subject your tendons to higher forces by doing exercises that are more strenuous. For example, imagine you've "only" been squatting 100 kg and then you decide to squat 150 kg. Alternatively, maybe you've been squatting 100 kg at a slow tempo and then you decide to go with a much faster tempo.

In both scenarios, the force on the patellar tendons increases dramatically from one training session to the next and because you haven't built the tensile strength of the tendons up over weeks, your tendons will not be able to cope with it. They will dip into reactive tendinopathy or worse, tendon dysrepair.

In the end, it's usually a combination of overtraining and too much too soon that leads to patellar tendonitis.

Chapter 4: How You Can Treat Patellar Tendonitis Successfully

This chapter outlines the 3-step process that is the minimal requirement for successfully treating patellar tendonitis. The first step is to stop the overuse of the patellar tendon and to give your knees ample time to recover after exercise. Rest does not mean a complete cessation of all activities, however, and I discuss what training can still be done while you heal. The second step is to start the healing process of your patellar tendon by performing special exercises; the science behind these exercises is presented here, and the technique is introduced. A more detailed description is given in chapter five. The third and last step entails fixing the factors that contribute to the overload of the patellar tendon. This involves using the stretching, massage, strengthening and mobility techniques given in chapter five to address the underlying factors.

Your Most Important Step

Several research studies have confirmed that you cannot recover from chronic patellar tendonitis if you're still playing your sport at the previous level (Visnes et al. 2005; Visnes, Bahr 2007). Hence, the most important step for fixing jumper's knee is stopping all activities that cause or increase pain in your patellar tendon.

Chapter 2 introduced you to the tendinopathy continuum and based on that concept you can understand why giving your tendon enough time to repair after increased demands were placed on it is an absolute necessity. If you don't stop the activity that has damaged your patellar tendon, the cycle will continue and your tendon will inevitably become weaker.

I can't emphasize this enough: to treat jumper's knee successfully, you have to stop participating in the activities that overloaded your knees in the first place. Don't do any jumping or running and avoid all activities that place load on your knee while it's bent for a week or two.

The reason you're doing this is to establish a baseline level of pain. During this initial rest period, take note of how your pain changes. Write it down on a scale of 1 to 10 (10 being the worst pain you ever felt) in a small journal, together with the activities you did on that particular day. This information will be tremendously helpful for your recovery, as it enables you to identify the activities that overstress your knees.

During this initial rest period, you can already start the treatment program suggested in this book, with the exception of the squats. Once your pain doesn't decrease any further, you can start with the eccentric squats. At that point, the pain scores you've written down during the rest period can be used to modify the squat exercises. We'll talk about that in detail together with the technique description in a later chapter.

Remember: if you insist on training or competing with your injured knee, you will prevent healing. You're only allowed activities that don't cause or increase pain and you will track that with your journal.

It's like giving up immediate gratification for a reward that you'll get later. Once you've completed the training program, your knees will be healthier than before and you'll be able to set new records. However, if you keep sabotaging your healing you won't get back to 100% and you'll struggle with frequent setbacks.

If you don't believe how serious patellar tendonitis can become, just go to Google and search for "patellar tendonitis years". You'll find countless stories about people who struggled with it for years. At least one long-term study has shown that even after 15 years, symptoms can persist to a certain degree (Kettunen et al. 2002).

The longer you wait with taking action, the weaker your tendon will become and the more treatment time the injury will take. Additionally, a weaker tendon is more likely to tear, which would require an expensive surgery and many months of rehab.

Jumper's knee is a serious injury and requires a serious commitment on your part if you want to beat it, so do yourself a favor and don't gamble on your long-term health for some short-term fun. Stay away from sports as long as it takes to get your knees healthy again.

How You Can Continue Training In Spite of Patellar Tendonitis

Patellar tendonitis is all about the load placed on your patellar tendon. You can significantly reduce the load on your tendon by fixing the contributing factors mentioned in the previous chapter, which may already reduce the load on your knees enough to allow you to continue your training. However, if you find that your pain still increases after training you need to take some additional steps.

If you've improved your movement technique for jumping and running as much as possible, the only other way to take load off your knees is by omitting jumping and explosive activities. I know from experience that most athletes frown upon the idea of doing less, but there's one thing you need to understand. Chances are you have developed jumper's knee because you're already stronger and more explosive than your teammates and opposing players. In other words, strength and explosiveness aren't your weaknesses!

However, all athletes have weaknesses and if it's not strength, chances are it's something else. Maybe your technique could use some practice (yes, we're talking about practice) or maybe your understanding of the game needs some improvement. Be this as it may, you can always find a way to elevate your game in spite of certain handicaps, you just need to identify your weaknesses and improve them.

By working on your weaknesses, your overall value as a player improves much faster than by working on your strengths. Improving your strengths further takes much more time and yields a smaller overall return of investment.

My Personal Experience with Skill and Strength

Back when I played basketball in our university league, I quickly discovered that the easiest way for me to become better was to get stronger and more explosive. Very few of the athletes in that league did weightlifting, which is why a mere 8 weeks of strength training could already give you a huge competitive advantage.

Additionally, being 6'6" (1.98 m) and weighing 161 pounds (73 kg) you could definitely say that strength and explosiveness were weaknesses of mine.

Many of the other athletes in that league had started playing basketball at a very young age. Their ball handling and technique were at a level that was difficult for me to attain, as I had only started playing basketball a few years prior.

I had over 15 years of volleyball training under my belt, but that had little carry-over to dribbling, shooting, and other basketball-specific movements. Getting stronger was the most effective way to gain an advantage over these more experienced players.

Soon I was able to jump higher than everyone else could, giving me a much better chance to grab a rebound for example. Of course, I also kept playing at the same weekly volume as my explosiveness went up and I didn't think anything of it. Sadly, a few months down the road, my dominant leg had become a bit achy and in retrospect, it makes perfect sense why I was one of the few who developed jumper's knee.

My teammates spent as much time playing as I did. However, my force output was higher than theirs and I think it's also safe to say that as a center/power forward you jump more often than someone who plays guard.

My knees just couldn't keep up with the increased load. If you combine strength training with an explosive sport such as volleyball or basketball, it's easy to slip into overloading your knees, especially if you don't know the first thing about jumping technique and back then, I didn't.

Once I had become stronger, the most effective way for me to take load off my knees was to improve my technique (e.g., jump shot and post-up game), so that there would be no need to go for offensive rebounds, thereby lowering the number of jumps per game.

This story illustrates how I turned strength and explosiveness from a weakness into a strong point, but then made the mistake of placing too much training time on this already strong aspect of my game. I neglected technique, thinking that I wouldn't be able to compete on technique with the more experienced players. It took me a long time to realize that spending less time on strength training and more time on technique would have made me a more formidable opponent.

I still needed to work on my weak patellar tendons and that's when I first looked into treatment exercises for jumper's knee.

The Most Effective, Research-Based Treatment Exercise

Eccentric exercises were mentioned in research as a way to resolve chronic tendonitis as early as 1986 (Stanish et al. 1986), but it wasn't until the land-mark study done by Alfredson in 1998 that eccentrics slowly became more widely known as an effective treatment approach for tendinosis (Alfredson et al. 1998).

Alfredson subjected 15 recreational athletes suffering from Achilles tendinopathy to a 12-week program of heavy-load eccentric calf training. Before the intervention, all of the participants had suffered chronic pain that prevented them from running. After going through the eccentric training for 12 weeks, all of the 15 participants were able to run again and pain was reduced significantly.

A control group of 15 athletes with the same background and similar symptoms was treated conventionally (i.e., rest, different footwear, NSAIDs, physical therapy). Conventional treatment was unsuccessful for all of these athletes and they all had to undergo surgery eventually.

The eccentric exercises used to heal tendinosis required the athlete to extend the muscle with the injured tendon slowly under load. For Achilles tendinopathy, this meant doing calf exercises that placed more load on the lowering portion of the movement and lowering the weight slowly under control.

The same concept can be applied to the patellar tendon by squatting with a higher eccentric load on the patellar tendon (i.e. by doing eccentric squats). To increase the load on the patellar tendon, a 25-

degree slanted board should be used (Purdam et al. 2003; Purdam 2004).

Researchers have tested eccentric squats on a decline board against a number of other exercise modalities to treat patellar tendinosis. Eccentric squats have been compared with regular bodyweight squats that placed equal emphasis on the eccentric as well as the concentric component (Jonsson 2005), with eccentric squats on a flat surface (Purdam 2004), and eccentric squats off a step (Young 2005). In each case, eccentric squats on a decline have been found superior in one or more ways, most notably when it came to pain reduction.

Performing eccentric exercises on a leg extension machine in conjunction with training on a hamstring curl machine has also been shown to reduce pain in athletes (Cannell 2001). Researchers compared the machine training to drop squats, a squat in which you rapidly lower yourself into a squat position, thus placing a lot of load on your patellar tendon. Cannell and colleagues found no significant statistical difference between the outcomes of both groups.

There are two reasons why I would consider eccentric squats on a decline superior to drop squats. The first is because drop squats only stress the patellar tendon at the point of return, the point at which you reach parallel, and not through the full range of motion like eccentric squats on a decline. Therefore, drop squats put more emphasis on certain parts of the tendon, but don't target the entire tendon.

The second reason why I'd take eccentric squats on a decline over drop squats is that drop squats do not allow as much control over the movement as decline eccentrics. Without as much control over the movement, you can't fine-tune the amount of load you place on your knees and it's easy to overstress your knees. Additionally, the ballistic nature of drop squats makes ingraining good movement technique more difficult. It's harder to prevent your knees from caving inward when you're doing ballistic movement than it is when you're moving slowly.

I would also prefer eccentric squats on a decline to leg extension and hamstring curls because access to special equipment is not always a given and can hinder adherence to a training protocol. Having easy access to a decline board and doing simple bodyweight exercises robs you of any excuses for not sticking with your training regimen. Moreover, these machine-based exercises are inferior to squatting when it comes to their functional outcome (i.e., how much better an athlete becomes) and their risk-to-benefit ratio (Cressey 2006).

To learn more about why using the leg extension machine is bad for your knees, check out the respective article I've linked to on the online resources page: http://www.fix-knee-pain.com/jumpers-knee-book-guide/

There are two criticisms that can be brought against eccentric squats on a decline board. First, if they are done with the knees coming forward, they place a lot of pressure on the patellar tendon and ingrain a movement pattern that increases your risk for patellar tendon overload in the future (e.g., when jumping with the knees coming forward). Second, squatting on a decline will mask limitations in ankle dorsiflexion range of motion.

To fix these shortcomings, squat with your shins close to vertical and do ankle dorsiflexion drills.

In summary, eccentric squats on a decline board are an effective treatment exercise for patellar tendinosis, the chronic injury stage, according to today's research. As explained before, you're in this chronic stage of patellar tendonitis if you've had pain for more than a few months.

If you haven't had pain for that long, simply giving your tendons enough time to recover after training and training only at an intensity that does not cause pain might allow your tendon to recover. You will use your pain scores to judge that. Additionally, you'll have to work on the factors that contribute to patellar tendonitis to ensure your tendons stay healthy in the future.

In short, if you're in the reactive tendinopathy/early dysrepair phase you modify your activity so that it doesn't cause or increase pain, and work on the contributing factors. If you're in the late dysrepair/degenerative tendinopathy phase you have to drop your activity, start doing eccentric exercises, and work on the contributing factors using the stretching and massage techniques, strengthening exercises, and mobility work discussed in the next chapter.

How to Do Eccentric Squats

For squats, the eccentric part is the part during which you lower your body. The lowering movement needs to be slow and steady. The descent should take around 3 to 5 seconds for each repetition. You can stand up at a faster speed than that, taking around two seconds to get up (the concentric part of squats).

During the eccentric, you place all your weight on your legs. During the concentric, you take some load off your legs by assisting yourself. How you assist yourself will depend on the equipment you have available.

The easiest option would be to place chairs on either side of the slanted board so that you can help yourself up by holding on to the chairs. You could also place the board in front of a door and pull yourself up on the door. The important thing is to place less weight on the legs when standing up.

If you're training one leg, you can shift most of your weight onto that one leg on the way down and then use both legs on the way up.

These technique questions will be discussed in detail in a later part of the book.

Chapter 5: Effective Healing Exercises for Jumper's Knee

In the previous chapters, you've learned about the cause of jumper's knee and about several important factors that contribute to it. We've also talked about an effective treatment exercise you can use to strengthen your patellar tendon. You now have all pieces of the puzzle in front of you, so it's time to put them together.

This chapter will first introduce you to the tools you need to complete the program. After that, we will talk about self-massage exercises for removing tension from your muscles without having to pay for an expensive massage. Next, I will introduce you to a couple of joint mobility exercises for jumper's knee. Lastly, we'll cover the strengthening exercises you will be doing.

The next chapter will show you how to put these exercises together into a treatment program for jumper's knee.

Essential Equipment: Cheap & Versatile

If you want to complete the treatment program successfully, you need to invest in a few pieces of equipment. Some of these tools you might already own and even if you don't, the equipment doesn't have to be expensive.

An overview of the mentioned pieces of equipment can be found here: http://www.fix-knee-pain.com/jumpers-knee-book-guide

Essential Piece of Equipment #1: Training Journal

You will use the training journal to write down your daily pain scores (scale of 1 to 10, 10 being the worst pain you ever felt) and to write down all relevant activities you did on a certain day. If you took a 5-mile hike, you'll write it down in your journal. If you did a training session of the treatment program, you'll write the exercises and repetitions down in the training journal.

At first glance, this may seem complicated, but it only takes a few seconds. This habit will help you stay on track and allows you to discover activities that influence your pain. Additionally, it's very satisfying to thumb through a journal that lists all the work you did for your health.

The training journal can be a nice notebook such as a Moleskine journal, but any type of notebook will do. Make sure it's on hand whenever you do the exercises.

Essential Piece of Equipment #2: Foam Roller

You will use the foam roller for the self-massage exercises. Foam rolling will help you remove soft-tissue restrictions from your fascia. These restrictions limit how well your muscles and tissues slide on top of each other and influence your flexibility, movement quality, and force output. Additionally, soft tissue limitations can cause pain.

Personally, I prefer using the RumbleRoller. It comes with small thorns that will dig into your fascia and allows you to hit parts of the muscle you might miss with a regular roller. However, if you don't want to spend money on a RumbleRoller, you can also get a regular foam roller.

Lastly, many gyms already have foam rollers, so maybe you don't need to buy one altogether. Just remember that equipment that is easily accessible in your home makes adherence to the training program more likely.

Essential Piece of Equipment #3: Slanted Board

You will stand on the slanted board for the eccentric squats. If you have some power tools you can easily build this yourself out of some leftover wood. You can access plans how to build a slanted board on the online resources page http://www.fix-knee-pain.com/jumpers-knee-book-guide

If you don't want to build the board yourself, you can buy one on Amazon or elsewhere on the web. Links are included on the online resources page as well. You can use the same board if you have Achilles tendonitis or if you just want to stretch your calves. These boxes are also called heel cord boxes.

Essential Piece of Equipment #4: Rubber Band

Elastic bands are one of the most versatile pieces of equipment you'll ever own. Among other things, you can use them for stretching, to increase the effectiveness of joint mobility exercises, and to strengthen your shoulders and rotator cuff.

In the patellar tendonitis program, we will use elastic bands to make certain exercises harder and to make ankle mobility drills more effective.

There are countless elastic bands on the market and it's tough to know which one to buy. Personally, I've used a green Theraband (5.5 meters long, that's about 18 feet) and then just looped it several times to get the resistance I needed. I've had this band for almost two years now, used it indoors and outdoors, and abused it many different ways. It's still in good condition. Alternatively, you can shop around for other bands.

If you don't want to spend money on a resistance band, you can use manual resistance for some of the exercises by using ankle weights or something similar, but it's not as convenient.

Self-Massage Exercises for Important Muscles

The premise of self-massage is simple: you apply massage to yourself by using a number of tools. This can be a tennis ball, a lacrosse ball, a wooden stick, a foam-roller or another useful device (*e.g.*, piece of PVC pipe or just your hand). By applying different amounts pressure to different regions of a muscle, you can find scar tissue, adhesions or trigger points based on where you're particularly sensitive.

By contracting and lengthening the muscle during the massage, more restrictions can be uncovered. You could use your hands to apply pressure with the tool, or you could use your bodyweight to create pressure by putting the tool on the ground and placing the body part you want to massage on top of it. Now roll back and forth. Hit every aspect of the muscle and try to release painful areas.

If you apply too much pressure or work on one area too long you are likely to do more harm than good, as you're actually causing more damage to the tissue. You have to apply a reasonable amount of pressure and how much that is exactly depends on your individual situation.

It should be uncomfortable, but not painful. Keep massaging a certain muscle until you feel like there is no more improvement to be had and then move on to the next muscle. You will derive more benefits from performing self-massage daily at a medium intensity than if you were to perform 2 sessions a week with high intensity.

What to Pay Attention to When Foam Rolling

Foam rolling should not be used on body parts that have recently been injured. You should consult your physician about foam rolling if you have circulatory problems or chronic pain conditions such as fibromyalgia.

Please also note that while foam rolling is a cheap and easy way to improve tissue quality, results will not appear overnight. You will have to work on your fascia daily for a week or more in order to notice improvements. With foam rolling you're only targeting your soft-tissue (i.e., you should not be rolling your joints or other bony structures).

The pressure you create with the roller shouldn't cause pain, but needs to be great enough to be effective. Just imagine you're getting a massage: you wouldn't want the therapist to leave bruises, but you don't want them to be too gentle either.

In time, tissue quality will improve and you can spend less time foam rolling; but in the beginning, you might have to spend between 1 to 2 minutes per muscle to achieve results. Don't roll a muscle longer than that, as it can actually have a negative impact on tissue quality.

If you want to do more, just do several sessions per day. Once you've done this for a couple of weeks you will know when you've reached the point of diminishing returns.

List of Self-Massage Exercises

The following pages contain a list of self-massage exercises that are important for dealing with patellar tendonitis. You can do them in any order you like, but working neighboring muscle groups in a sequence saves some time.

Adductors

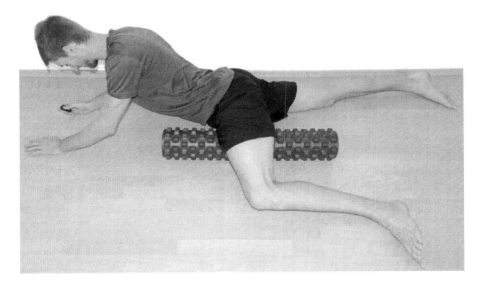

Foam rolling the adductors can be a bit awkward. However, this is an important muscle group, which is why you need to take care of it.

Purpose

Improve soft-tissue quality in the adductors. Tight adductors pull your knees inward and increase your chances of knee injury.

Setup

Lie down on your stomach and put one leg out to the side. Place the foam-roller on the inside of the thigh of that leg. Roll by moving your hip from side to side.

How to Perform

Supporting your bodyweight with your hands, place pressure on the area in contact with the foam-roller and gently roll the muscle. Bend and straighten the knee of the leg you're working to hit different muscles and reveal more restrictions.

Common Mistakes

Sitting with your legs crossed during the day shortens your adductors over time. Getting rid of this habit can be difficult, but it's worth it in the end.

Regressions

To decrease pressure on the adductors you put more weight on the hands and the bottom leg.

Calves

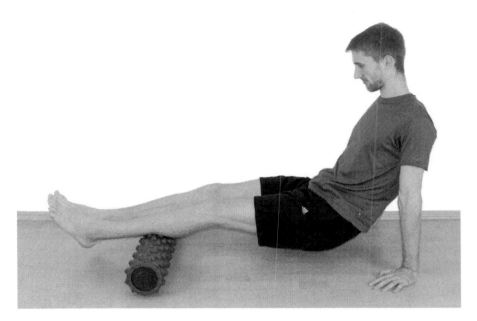

The calves have very high endurance and are essential for upright gait. Factors such as improper footwear and unbalanced training protocols (*i.e.,* lots of plantarflexion, but no dorsiflexion) can influence the soft-tissue quality of the calves. Depending on how much you have neglected your calves this area might be particularly painful. Remember not to overdo it and to use a reasonable amount of pressure.

Purpose

Improve soft-tissue quality of the calves. Tight calves will make completely straightening your knee harder and thus contribute to overload of the patellar tendon. Additionally, tightness in the calves can lead to plantar fasciitis.

Setup

Place the foam-roller under one or both calves.

How to Perform

Support your bodyweight with your hands and roll the calf muscle. Work all sides of the calves by pointing your knee(s) completely to the left, diagonally to the left, to the top, diagonally to the right, and completely to the right. You can improve the efficacy of this exercise further by flexing and extending your feet as well as bending and straightening your knees during the massage. Don't forget to hit the Achilles tendon as well.

Common Mistakes

Using too much pressure will create additional adhesions between muscles. More isn't better with foam rolling. Instead of using too much pressure just roll more often to make quicker progress.

Regressions

If rolling both calves at the same time is still too hard for you, you could try rolling just one calf and supporting more weight with the other leg. You can also massage your calves using a tennis ball in your hand, which allows for a more precise application of pressure.

Progressions

To increase pressure you can place one leg on the other, use a tennis ball on the ground, or have a partner perform the massage on your calves using a stick. Certain trigger points can only be found with smaller implements, so be sure to try these suggestions at some point.

Foot, Underside

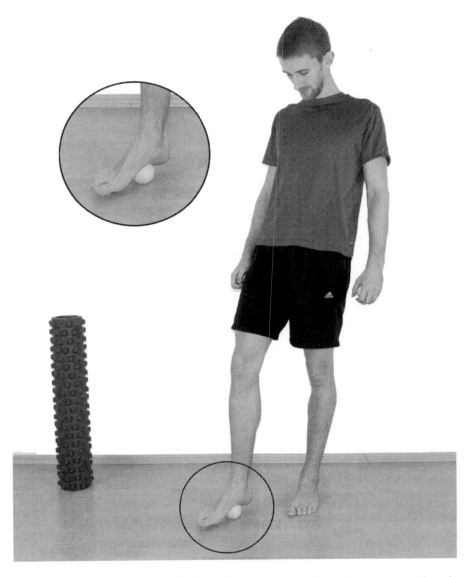

The fascia of the whole body is interconnected and one area that is sometimes forgotten during treatment is the underside of your foot. However, this small area can have a big impact on your flexibility. For example, massaging this area can increase your range of motion in the toe touch noticeably. Try it: test your toe touch ROM, then do this massage on both feet, and then retest the ROM.

Purpose

Foam rolling the underside of the foot aims to release soft-tissue restrictions of the plantar fascia.

Setup

Place a tennis or lacrosse ball under your foot.

How to Perform

Roll the underside of your foot.

Regressions

Decrease the amount of pressure on your foot by placing more weight on the supporting leg.

Progressions

To increase pressure you can use a smaller implement or increase the force. However, I recommend you take a barefoot walk over a path with lots of pebbles of different sizes. This will give your feet an intense massage and you can feel the improve blood circulation hours after you've returned from your walk.

Gluteus Maximus

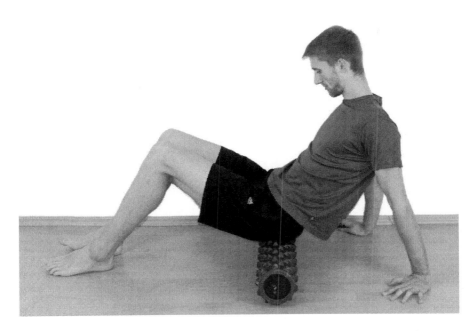

Long periods spent sitting will cause the layers of fascia in your buttocks to laminate together, thereby contributing to the problems many people have with using their glutes. Make sure to roll your gluteus maximus thoroughly to reveal and resolve any soft-tissue problems in that area.

Purpose

Improve soft-tissue quality in the gluteus maximus to increase hip strength and motor control of the thigh (and thus the knee). Releasing tension in the gluteus maximus, as it could cause lower back and lateral knee pain.

Setup

Sit down on the foam-roller, supporting your weight with your hands behind your back.

How to Perform

Roll your buttocks and straighten as well as extend your hips throughout the drill to search for more soft-tissue restrictions.

Regressions

Place more weight on your hands to decrease pressure on your glutes.

Progressions

To increase pressure on your glutes you can roll one side at a time or use a smaller implement such as a tennis ball. However, I have found this exercise hard to perform with a tennis ball and prefer to use the RumbleRoller.

Gluteus Medius

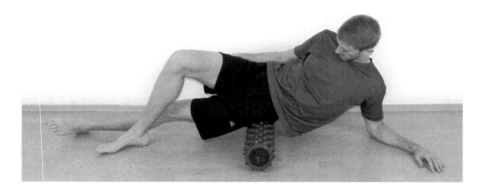

Purpose

Improve soft-tissue quality of Gluteus Medius to increase movement control of the thigh.

Setup

Lie down on your side and place the roller under your hip, slightly towards your back. Support your weight with the elbow of the bottom arm, the hand of the top arm, and the non-working leg.

How to Perform

Roll the muscles on the outside of your hip and try to hit those that are towards the back by rotating your hip slightly upwards.

Common Mistakes

The area you're targeting lies under the hip bones you can feel on either side of your hip and slightly to the back. Don't roll those hip bones.

Regressions

Decrease pressure by placing more weight on your supporting limbs or massage the area with a stick to allow for even finer control of the pressure.

Progressions

To increase pressure you can take the bottom leg off the floor or use a smaller implement. Having a partner massage the area with a stick can also be beneficial.

Hamstrings

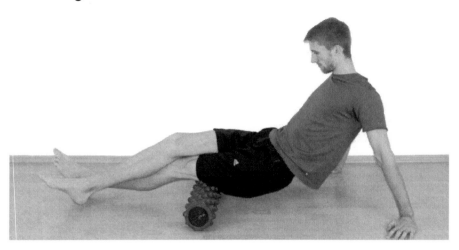

The hamstrings can develop soft-tissue problems due to overuse or strains. Such issues will decrease tissue extensibility and can potentially lead to pain behind your knee.

Purpose

Resolving soft-tissue problems in the hamstrings will provide several benefits such as improved hip mobility into hip flexion and higher athletic performance.

Setup

Place the roller under one or both thighs.

How to Perform

Roll the underside of your thighs, starting from the area close to your hip. Remember to roll the area slightly from either side to hit all muscles in this group. Additionally, try to flex and extend the knee during the massage.

Common Mistakes

Tensing the hamstrings during the massage will make the drill less efficient. Relax the working leg as much as possible to derive maximum benefit.

Regressions

To apply less pressure you can either roll both legs or place one leg on the ground and put more weight on this additional supporting limb.

Progressions

You can increase the pressure by placing just one thigh on the roller and having the other leg up in the air or even stacked on top the working leg. Increase the pressure further by working with a smaller implement or by having a partner perform the massage with a stick.

Iliotibial Band

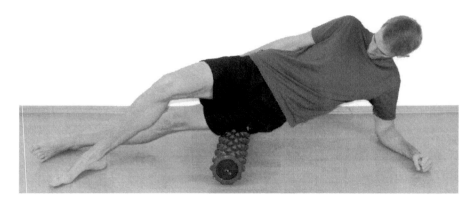

The IT band is an important stabilizing structure for your knee. Whether or not foam rolling the IT band delivers benefits is a controversial topic, but since many people say it helped them I included it.

Purpose

Too much tension in the IT band can result in a sudden onset of pain on the outside of your knee.

Setup

Lie down on your side and place the roller on the outside of your bottom thigh. Support your weight with the non-working limbs.

How to Perform

Roll up and down your thigh in smaller strokes, starting from the top of the thigh. With the IT band, I've found massage with the stick and the tennis ball particularly useful, as these implements allow you to penetrate deeper into the tissue.

Common Mistakes

Don't roll the bony prominences around your hip and your knee. Concentrate on the soft-tissue.

Regressions

Place more weight on supporting limbs.

Progressions

Use a smaller implement or stack your legs on top of each other.

Quadriceps: Rectus Femoris

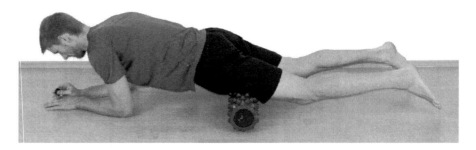

The Rectus Femoris crosses both, the knee and the hip, and usually has soft-tissue restrictions leading to less extensibility, which tilts the pelvis of the person forward.

Purpose

Releasing tension in the Rectus Femoris can "feed slack" to the patellar tendon and speed up recovery from patellar tendonitis. It will also help to improve your posture.

Setup

Lie down on your stomach and place the roller on the front of your thighs.

How to Perform

Roll the front of your thighs in small strokes, starting from the area close to your hip. Roll the entire length of your thigh once and then repeat with flexed knees.

Common Mistakes

Make sure to maintain proper spinal alignment by engaging your abs and your glutes. Do not let your lower back sag down.

Regressions

You can reduce the pressure by partly supporting your weight on your toes or by massaging the Rectus Femoris with a stick instead.

Progressions

Roll only one leg at a time or use a smaller implement to increase pressure.

Quadriceps: Vastus Lateralis

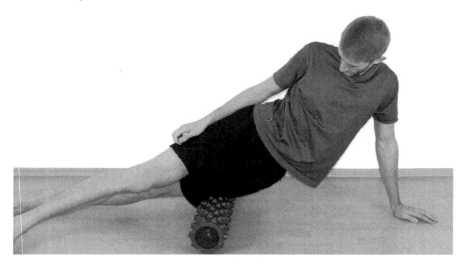

Purpose

You foam-roll the Vastus Lateralis to remove potential adhesions between the Vastus Lateralis and the Iliotibial Band, as well as to release tension from the Vastus Lateralis. Both can contribute to pain on the outside of your knee, patellar-tracking problems, and limit your performance.

Setup

Lie down on your side and place the roller under the outside of your thigh, slightly to the front.

How to Perform

Roll the Vastus Lateralis in small strokes, starting from the area close to your hip. Flex and extend the knee to reveal more soft-tissue problems.

Common Mistakes

If you roll too much on the side of your thigh, you will mostly hit the

Iliotibial Band.

Regressions

Place more weight on the supporting limbs to decrease pressure. If that's still too much pressure, you can opt for a massage with the stick instead.

Progressions

Stack the non-working leg on top of the bottom leg to increase tension or use a smaller implement.

Quadriceps: Vastus Medialis

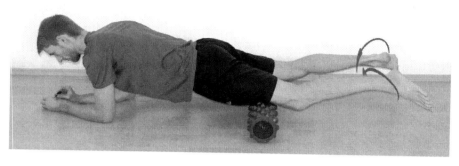

Soft-tissue problems in the Vastus Medialis can lead to this muscle group "shutting down". In combination with people's general fear of squatting and squatting deep in particular, this leads to a very weak Vastus Medialis, which contributes to the patella tracking slightly to the outside.

Purpose

Remove soft-tissue restrictions in the Vastus Medialis.

Setup

Lie down on your stomach and place the roller on the front of your thighs. Point your knees to the outside to hit the Vastus Medialis.

How to Perform

Gently roll back and forth while putting pressure on the inside front portion of your thigh.

Common Mistakes

Rolling the knee or rolling too far on the inside of the thigh.

Regressions

Massage the area with the stick to be able to use less pressure.

Progressions

Roll only one leg to increase the pressure on the target area.

Tensor Fascia Latae

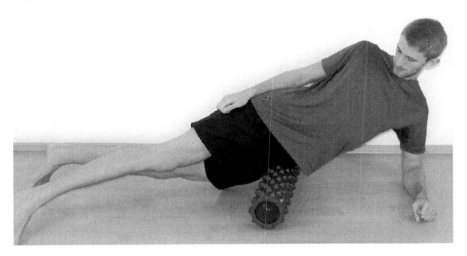

Purpose

Release tension in the TFL, as this tension can contribute to Iliotibial Band Syndrome and generally decreases movement quality.

Setup

Lie down on your side and place the roller just below the bony prominence on the side of your hip.

How to Perform

Roll the area gently and slightly tilt your body to the front and to the back in order to hit the target muscle from more angles.

Regressions

You can place more weight on the supporting limbs to reduce pressure on the target area. If that is still too much pressure, you can also opt to massage the TFL with a stick instead.

Progressions

To use more pressure you can stack your legs on top of each other or use a smaller implement. Additionally, performing the massage with the stick can reveal more soft-tissue problems.

Patellar Tendonitis Joint Mobility Exercises

Joint mobility exercises provide numerous benefits. They help supply the cartilage of the joint with nutrients, aid in restoring range of motion in the joint, help us improve motor control and strengthen our ligaments and joints, thereby decreasing the chance of injury. Additionally, joint mobility releases muscle tension.

The following joint mobility exercises are particularly useful when you want to prevent patellar tendonitis.

Heel Circles

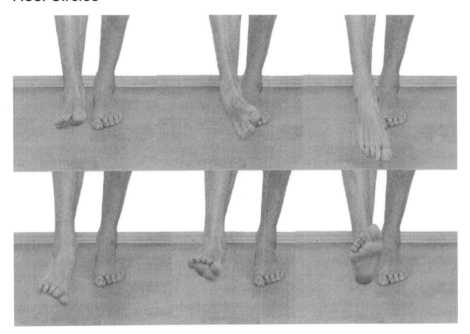

Purpose

Mobilize the ankle in all directions without applying external load by just using your own strength. Strengthening the muscles that create ankle dorsiflexion.

Setup

Stand on one foot and place the other foot slightly in front of you. This exercise can also be performed when sitting or lying on the ground.

How to Perform

Draw circles with the heel of your working foot. Increase the size of the circles as much as possible.

Common Mistakes

By concentrating on the movement of the heel instead of the movement of the toes, the exercise becomes more efficient.

Regressions

If you have pain in certain ranges of motion, you work in the pain-free ranges of motion.

Progressions

The goal of this exercise is to mobilize without load, which is why there is no progression.

Dorsiflexion Drill

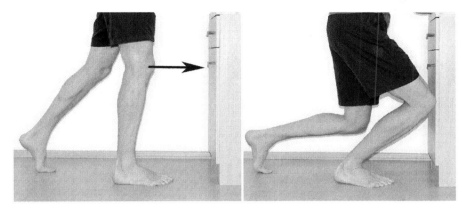

Purpose

Improve ankle range of motion.

Setup

Position yourself in front of a wall or a piece of furniture.

How to Perform

Keeping your heel planted you let your knee come forward to touch the object and then return to the starting position. Slide your foot back a bit if you've consistently managed to touch the object without straining. Compare range of motion between both legs and work more on the ankle with less ROM.

If your calves are very tight, you might feel a light stretch in the bottom portion of the calf of the working leg.

You can make this more effective by having your working knee trace a half circle to the outside of your body. For a more detailed description, check out my free email series on the most common causes for knee pain: http://www.fix-knee-pain.com/jumpers-knee-book-guide/

Common Mistakes

Don't let the arches of your feet collapse and don't have your knee move to the midline of the body. Keep your feet pointing straight ahead and your knee tracking over your second toe.

Regressions

If pain keeps you from increasing your range of motion, you can try the Soleus stretch with a band.

Progressions

You can move your knee in circles over the outside front of your foot. You can also carefully lift the supporting leg off the floor to put even more weight on the ankle.

Stepping Over the Fence

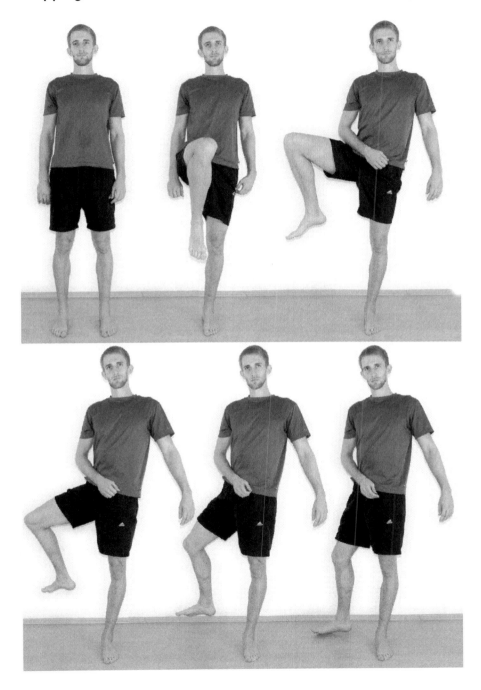

Purpose

This drill improves balance, hip mobility and strength, as well as coordination.

Setup

Stand with your feet underneath your hips and pointing forward.

How to Perform

Imagine you're standing with your side to a fence and you want to step over it. Keeping the rest of your body as motionless as possible, you pull one knee up as high as you can in front of your body. Holding that height you rotate that leg out as far as possible and once you can go any further you bring the foot of that leg down to gently touch the ground behind you. Now reverse the movement by tracing your steps back.

Common Mistakes

This should be a controlled movement and as such, you must not use momentum to complete the drill. It's ok to catch your balance if you fall, but try to stay in control.

Regressions

You may hold on to something for balance in the beginning, but wean yourself off quickly.

Progressions

Perform this drill by stepping over the back of a chair for a challenge.

Z-Sit

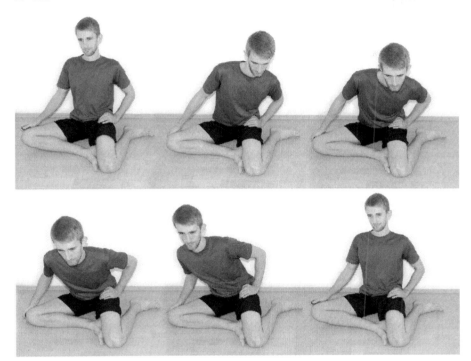

Purpose

Improve hip mobility and release tension from the hip muscles.

Setup

Sit down on the ground with your legs bent at a 45-degree angle. Bring both knees to the ground in the same direction, so that the foot of the outside knee touches the thigh of the other leg right above the knee.

How to Perform

Gently rotate your body while keeping your legs on the ground. After a certain number of repetitions, you can rotate your body in the other direction, after which you change the direction in which your legs are pointing and repeat the drill. Switch after you've released the tension in your hip.

Jumper's Knee Stretches

The following stretches will help you relieve tension from the patellar tendon. As you've learned earlier, if certain muscles are tight, the risk for developing patellar tendonitis increases, so be sure to do these stretches regularly. For best results, you should do them at least twice per day.

You can make these stretches more effective by using two techniques. In the first technique, you try to push yourself into the stretch actively, tensing the antagonist muscle of the one you want to stretch. For example, when stretching the calves by standing on a step you'd pull your feet up towards your knees to intensify the stretch.

The second technique requires the opposite movement. You resist the stretch for at least 5 seconds by creating tension in the muscle you want to stretch. When stretching your quadriceps for example, you'd try to extend your knee against the resistance of your hand.

Once you've created a lot of tension in the muscle for at least 5 seconds you release the tension, let out and audible sigh, and relax deeper into the stretch. The audible sigh is important, as it helps signal your muscles to relax.

Do each stretch for a total time of at least two minutes per side. Some people prefer to do all that time in one single set, others found dividing the total time into several sets to be more effective. Experiment and find what works best for you.

When Not to Stretch

Stretching messes with your body awareness and puts you at an increased risk of injury should you compete after having stretched. You can tell this is happening if you try to walk after having stretched your hamstrings or quadriceps for example. You can still walk, but something feels off.

Never stretch directly before a game or before your training. If you need to stretch to be able to get into certain positions in your sport, you obviously need to stretch more often, but not right before your competition.

List of Stretches

Calf Stretch

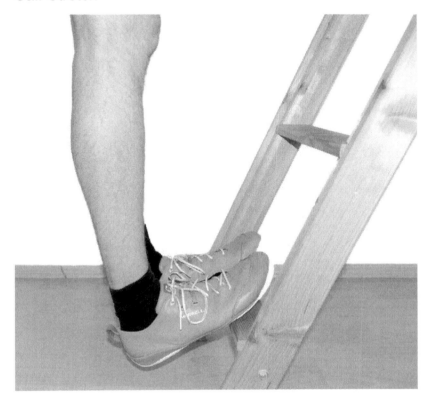

Purpose

Increasing extensibility of the Gastrocnemius improves ankle range of motion and reduces stress on structures on the front of the knee, as a tight Gastrocnemius would work against your quads in knee extension.

Setup

To stretch both calves at the same time, you place the balls of your feet on a stair and let your heels sink down.

How to Perform

Let the heels of your feet sink down and either actively pull your toes towards your knee or perform calf raises while letting your heels sink deeper into the stretch on the bottom part of the movement. Since the calves have a lot of endurance, it will be easier to use the first stretching method.

You should feel the stretch in your calves. Do this stretch with your knees straight and a little bent.

Common Mistakes

Don't let your ankles roll inwards. The same movement occurs when you intentionally over-pronate and let your feet become flat-footed.

Progressions

Perform the one-legged version of this stretch once you feel like the two-legged version provides no further benefit.

Hamstring Stretch

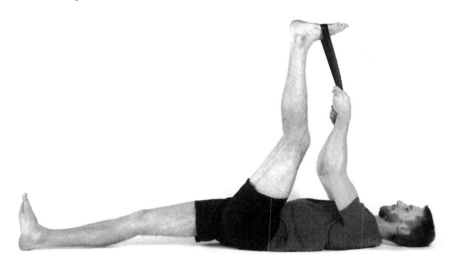

Purpose

The goal of this stretch is to reprogram the central nervous system to allow for more hamstring extensibility.

Setup

Lie on your back and make sure the curve in your lower back is not too big. You should be able to slide some fingers through, but not your whole hand.

Grab a strong elastic band, a belt, or a piece of rope, and sling it around your foot.

How to Perform

Raise your leg up as far as you can, until you feel a stretch in your hamstrings. Next, pull with your hands on the band as hard as you can and resist that tension with your leg. Imagine you're trying to push the foot of the working leg towards the other foot. Hold this tension for at least 5 seconds.

Let out an audible sigh and relax your hamstrings and arms for a second. Next, pull your leg closer to your chest until you feel tension in your hamstrings again. Now, pull as hard as you can on the band again and resist that tension. Go through this procedure until you can no longer go deeper into the stretch.

Make sure you perform this stretching series with your leg straight and with your leg bent at the knee. For the second position, setup with your knee as close to your chest as possible and then repeat the stretching steps.

Common Mistakes

Don't bend at the lower back. Make sure the distance between your lower back and the ground stays the same. If you can't maintain that distance, put a towel under your lower back.

Alternatives

The one-legged Romanian Deadlifts you will learn in the subchapter on strengthening exercises fulfill a similar purpose.

Hip Flexor Stretch with Wall Hold

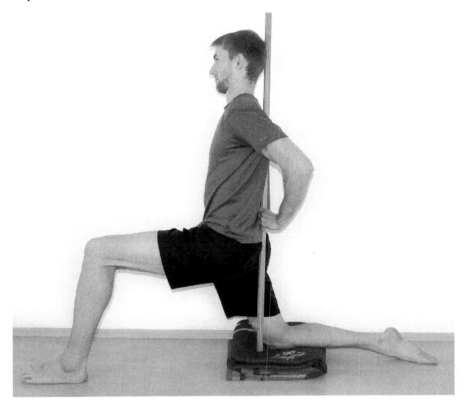

Purpose

Testing whether the hip flexor is weak, strengthening it, and increasing its extensibility.

Before You Begin

Before performing the stretch for the first time, perform the wall hold to test for hip flexor weakness. With your back to a wall, you stand on one foot while elevating the knee of the other leg to above hip level. The foot of the supporting leg can be a couple of inches away from the wall.

If you can hold this position for at least 30 seconds, your hip flexors are not weak. Should your hip flexors test weak, you will have to strengthen them by performing the wall hold before doing the stretches.

How to Perform

Get down in a lunge position with one knee on the ground. Make sure you have ample padding under your knee, by using something like a folded blanket or a pillow. Now squeeze the glute of the rear leg and imagine driving the knee back and into the ground, while having the hip sink down and forward.

Brace your abs, as if you're bracing for a punch. Don't let your abs protrude outwards, but work to stabilize your pelvis with your core musculature.

Personally, I prefer moving my rear leg back as I go deeper into the stretch, but you can also keep both feet stationary and just let the hip sink down and forward. You must not lean forward or let your back round.

You can place one hand at the lower back, so that you can tell how well you're contracting the glute. If you can't tell whether the curve in your lower back increases you can use a stick (see picture).

To increase the stretch even further, you can take the arm on the side of the working leg and reach over the opposite shoulder.

You should feel the stretch on the front of the hip of the working leg.

Common Mistakes

- Hunching over or leaning forward
- Letting the hip tilt forward (increased curve in the lower back)
- Relaxing the abs
- Relaxing the glutes of the working leg

Regressions

If you can't do this stretch because of pain or other reasons, check out my page on hip flexor stretches for alternative versions:

http://www.fix-knee-pain.com/psoas-stretch/

Progressions

Once your hip flexor extensibility and strength has increased, you can progress to the quadriceps stretch.

Quadriceps Stretch

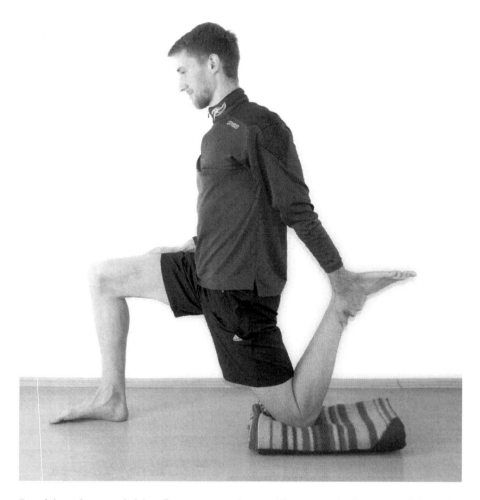

In this advanced hip flexor stretch you'll not only be stretching the Iliopsoas, but the Rectus Femoris as well.

Purpose

With this drill, we increase extensibility of the hip flexors and learn the difference between movement at the lower back and movement at the hip.

Setup

Assume a lunge position with the knee of the rear leg under your hip. Put some padding under the rear leg to protect it from the hard ground.

How to Perform

First you reach back to grab the ankle of the rear leg and pull it towards your buttocks. Getting into this position can be tricky, so hold on to something for balance if you have to. Make sure to find a position that is comfortable for your knee. Now you squeeze the abs and tense the glutes of the working leg. Remember to maintain a neutral spine and not to let your hip tilt forward (same alignment as in previous stretch). Push your hip forward and pull the ankle closer to your hip to increase the stretch.

To increase the efficiency of this stretch you can resist the stretch by pushing your foot against the resistance of your hand. After tensing up like that for 5 to 10 seconds, you relax deeper into the stretch. A thorough soft-tissue massage of the quadriceps is also highly recommended and it will make the stretch easier.

You should feel the stretch in the thigh of your working leg and in the front of the hip.

Common Mistakes

- Hunching over or leaning forward
- Letting the hip tilt forward (increased curve in the lower back)
- Relaxing the abs
- Relaxing the glutes of the working leg

Regressions

If this stretch is too tough for you, just perform the regular hip flexor stretch instead and advance later once you've gotten used to it.

Progressions

You can use an elastic band that pulls your hip forward to increase the intensity of the stretch even further. Loop it around the upper part of the working leg's thigh.

Strengthening Exercises

The following strengthening exercises will help you fix the factors that contribute to patellar tendonitis. However, to create good movement you also need to practice moving with good technique. Once your muscles are strong enough to maintain good movement quality, you need to train your nervous system to be able to produce the desired movement in your sport.

You could say that the strengthening exercises will help you improve the hardware, but once that has happened you still need to update the software to achieve the desired result.

To derive the most benefits out of the standing exercises, you should do them without shoes or just wearing minimalist footwear. Socks work as well. This is because the cushioning of regular sneakers robs your body of the ground input and makes maintaining balance more difficult.

Abduction Drill

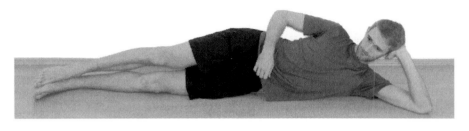

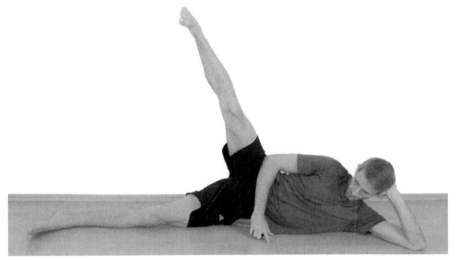

Purpose

This exercise specifically targets hip abduction strength.

Setup

Lie on your side and put some padding under your hip if you are on a hard surface. Keep your body in one line and stack both feet on top of each other.

How to Perform

Lift the upper leg up by moving solely from the hip. Keep the toes of the working **foot pointed towards the floor** to make sure you're using the right muscle groups. Lift the foot as high as you can and hold for a second. Then return to the starting position.

Don't worry if you don't have a lot range of motion in this exercise. Make sure to thoroughly foam-roll the muscles on the inside and on the outside of your thigh before commencing this exercise. Work to increase your ROM with every repetition.

Common Mistakes

- Holding your breath under exertion
- Rotating your foot out so that it is parallel to the ground or even pointing up (keep it pointing down)
- Moving your hip

Progressions

Perform this exercise with an elastic band wrapped around your legs ("Abduction Drill, with Band").

Abduction Drill, with Band

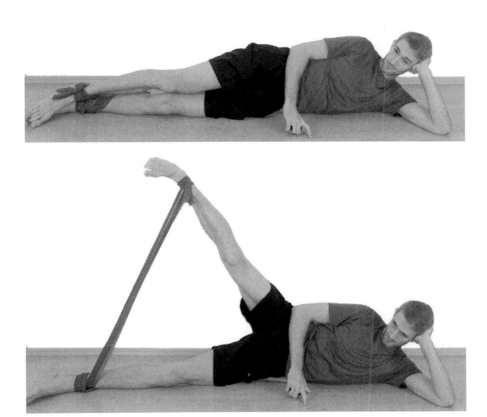

Purpose

This exercise specifically targets hip abduction strength and puts an additional resistance against the working muscle to increase its force output further.

Setup

Lie on your side and put some padding under your hip if you are on a hard surface. Wrap an elastic band around your feet. You can wrap it around the shinbones directly above your ankle or your thighs directly above the knee. The band should be extensible enough to allow you to perform the exercise in the full range of motion, so experiment with band length, strength, and placement to find the right combination. Keep your body in one line and stack both feet on top of each other.

How to perform

Lift the upper leg up by moving solely from the hip. Keep the toes of the working foot pointed towards the floor to make sure you're using the right muscle groups. Lift the foot as high as you can and hold for a second. Then return to the starting position.

Common Mistakes

- Holding your breath under exertion
- Using a band that is too short or too strong to allow full range of motion
- Rotating your foot out so that it is parallel to the ground or even pointing up (keep it pointing down)
- Moving your hip

Progressions

Contract the working muscle as much as possible in the top position and hold for up to 5 seconds.

Ankle Band Side Walk

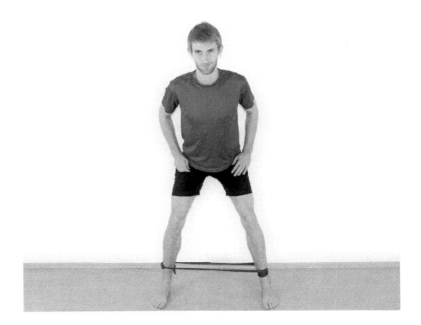

Purpose

Improve abduction strength of the hips and allow you to practice good movement technique under controlled load.

Setup

Take an elastic band and wrap it around your shins slightly above your ankles. Assume a half-squat position and have your feet slightly point towards the midline of your body. Stay on the balls of your feet during the exercise.

How to Perform

Leading with the heel, you take a controlled step out to the side. Next, you move the other foot to assume the half squat again in the new location. Move both feet in a controlled fashion and don't drag them on the floor.

Common Mistakes

- Dragging the feet
- Not leading with the heel
- Moving in a jerky fashion

Regressions

As a regression of this exercise, you can use a lighter band or split your total number of repetitions up over more sets.

Clams

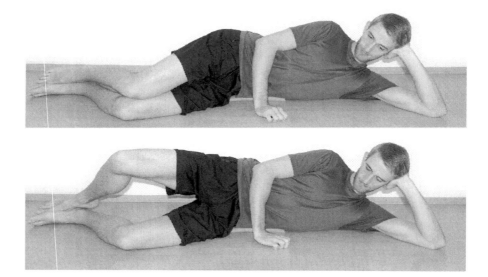

Purpose

Improve external rotation strength of the hips.

Setup

Lie down on your side and put some padding under your hip if you are on a hard surface. Bend your knees slightly and place them a bit in front of you.

How to Perform

Rotate the upper leg up by just using your hip muscles. Keep your feet relaxed throughout and don't push off with the toes. Keep your upper body and your hip stationary, only move the working leg. Hold the elevated position for a couple of seconds and then return to the starting position.

You should feel the exertion on the side of the hip.

Common Mistakes

- Tilting the hip back
- Holding your breath
- Pushing off with your foot

Regressions

It's ok if you have little range of motion in the beginning. Try to improve it gradually.

Progressions

Perform this exercise with an elastic band wrapped around your thighs just above your knees.

Clams, with Band

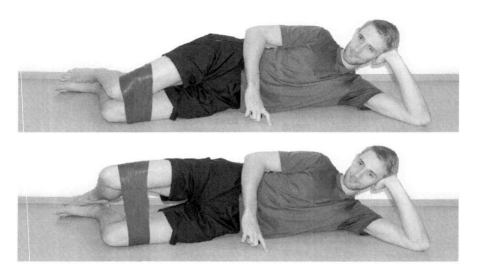

Purpose

Improve external rotation strength of the hips with additional resistance.

Setup

Lie down on your side and put some padding under your hip if you are on a hard surface. Bend your knees slightly and place them in front of you. Put an elastic band around your thighs just above your knees.

How to Perform

Rotate the upper leg up by just using your hip muscles. Keep your feet relaxed throughout and don't push off with the toes. Keep your upper body and your hip stationary, only move the working leg. Hold the elevated position for a couple of seconds and then return to the starting position. The exertion should be felt on the side of the hip.

With this variation, it's particularly important that you breathe normally throughout the exertion.

Common Mistakes

- Tilting the hip back
- Holding your breath
- Pushing off with your foot

Regressions

Perform the exercise without the elastic band.

Progressions

Use a stronger elastic band or hold the top position for up to 5 seconds. I've found that you don't really need a stronger band, as you can just tense the working muscles as much as possible once you've reached the point where you can't rotate out further.

Eccentric Squats on Slanted Board, Two Legs

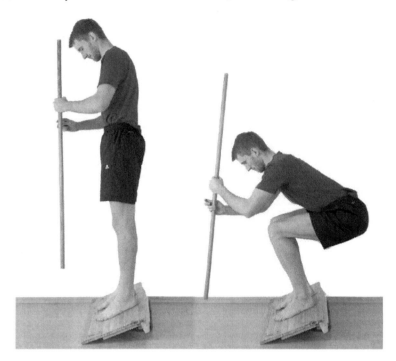

Purpose

The eccentric squat will increase collagen formation in your patellar tendon and helps restore good alignment to the collagen fibers.

Setup

Stand on a slanted board with your feet underneath your hips and pointing forward. Have something ready to assist yourself on the way up. I'm using a stick in the picture, but you could also place the board in front of an open door and hold onto the door handle. Alternatively, place some chairs next to the board to push off of on the way back up.

How to Perform

Lower yourself slowly, taking around 3 to 5 seconds, to the parallel

position. **The top of your thigh should be parallel to the ground.**
Next, take load off your knees by placing more weight on your support
(e.g., the stick, the chairs, the door handle) and return to the starting
position placing as little load as possible on your legs.

The proper squatting technique requires you to keep your shins as
close to vertical as possible. Sit your hips back as if you're reaching for
a chair that is far away. However, don't place your weight too far back,
as you can lose balance easily if you place all your weight on your heels.

Common Mistakes

- Making jerky movements (everything has to be smooth)
- Letting the knees come forward (keep your shins as close to vertical as possible)
- Letting the knees cave in or drift out (keep your knees above your toes)
- Moving with momentum

Alternative Variations

Squatting depth is a controversial subject among researchers and
professional trainers. An alternative variation of this drill has you move
through the full range of motion, so you lower yourself down until
your calves touch your hamstrings.

If you want to reclaim the full range of motion, as you should, start
going a little deeper with every training session. Remember to move
slowly.

Progressions

Place more weight on one leg on the way down to increase the load.
This will help you transition to the one-legged version of the drill.

Eccentric Squats on Slanted Board, One Leg

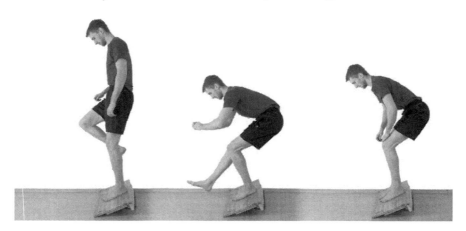

Purpose

The one-legged version places more load on your patellar tendon and helps you integrate the strength built through hip exercises into a movement that's closer to a real world scenario.

Setup

Stand on a slanted board with your feet underneath your hips and pointing forward.

How to Perform

Lift one foot off the ground, lower yourself slowly, and under control, until your quadriceps is parallel to the ground (notice how I haven't reached that depth yet in the second picture above). Take around 3 to 5 seconds for the way down.

The key is to move without momentum, as that prevents energy storage in your tendon.

Next, take load off your working leg, by placing the other foot on the ground again. Lift yourself up with both legs.

Common Mistakes

- Making jerky movements (everything has to be smooth)
- Letting the knee come forward (keep your shins as close to vertical as possible)
- Letting the knee cave in or drift out (keep your knees above your toes)
- Moving with momentum

While the one-legged squat will make your legs stronger (without increasing muscle mass), its main goal in our program is not that of strengthening your muscles. With this drill, we pursue two main goals.

One, we want to strengthen the patellar tendon and improve collagen alignment, thereby increasing tensile strength and two, we want to improve motor control by integrating the strength built through the other exercises into a good movement pattern.

Never think of single-leg squats as "working out". It's always movement practice, and never "working out". If you find you can't maintain good movement quality anymore, you need to stop. This is important because your motor control center will store every sloppy repetition as an "ok way to do it".

Once you actually depend on your muscle memory to bail you out, say when you've been running and jumping for an hour or more, you will rely on that muscle memory to prevent injuries. If you've stored countless crappy repetitions in your movement database, you will automatically return to that crappy way of moving. That's how injuries happen.

Again, this is movement practice, not working out.

Alternative Variations

This exercise can also be performed on even ground, which makes it a perfect drill to practice anywhere at any time.

Progressions

If you are pain-free in the one-legged squat to parallel just doing the eccentric, you can slowly go deeper with each session until you're doing the full range of motion single-leg squat. Be advised, however, that this is a very controversial exercise; while it's safe to perform if you've slowly eased into it over many weeks, you can be injured if you jump into the deep end of the pool too soon.

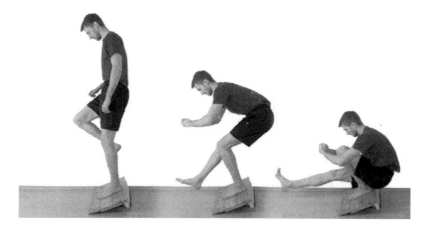

This exercise becomes stressful on the knees if you move with momentum and try to bounce yourself up. Once you start bouncing and moving with momentum you will use your tendon for energy storage, which increases the load on it. This increased load might cause you to relapse. Move slowly and under full control.

An alternative way you can progress this exercise is by doing both the concentric and eccentric part of the movement on one leg, but just going to parallel. It's a regular single-leg squat to parallel, only that you're still moving slowly.

With this variation, take around 3 to 5 seconds on the way down and around 3 seconds on the way up. We still want to avoid energy storage in the patellar tendon, which is why moving without momentum is very important.

Glute Bridge, Two Legs

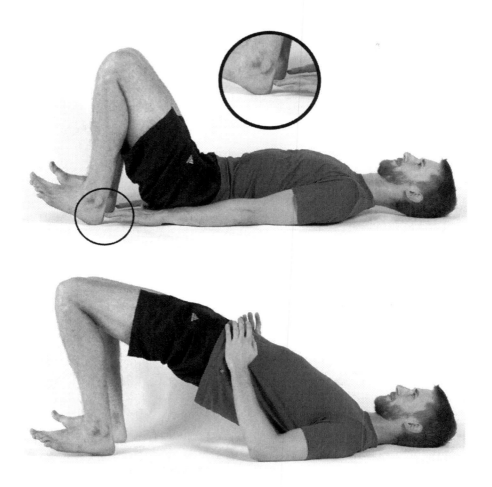

Purpose

The Glute Bridge improves gluteal activation and strength.

Setup

Lie down on your back and place your arms at your side. Bring your heels back towards your hip so that your fingertips touch your heels.

How to Perform

Lift your toes off the ground so that only your heel is touching the floor. Now, lift your hips up as high as you can. Check your hamstrings and your glutes with your hand for tension: your glutes should be much tenser than your hamstrings. Continue tensing your glutes in an effort to lift your hips higher and hold this position for a couple of seconds. Then come down, relax, and repeat.

Common Mistakes

Make sure that you're really tensing the glutes hard throughout the exercise and try to relax the hamstrings as much as possible. Touch the muscles with your hand to feel how tense they are. Don't let your toes come down. Keep pulling your toes up as high as you can.

Regressions

If you're having trouble isolating your glutes from your hamstrings, do prone hip extensions: lie down on your stomach, fold your legs at your knees to have 90-degree angle between your thighbone and shinbone. Now, lift one leg off the floor by contracting the buttocks muscles of that leg. Touch the muscles to make sure that you're only contracting the gluteal muscles and not your hamstrings.

Progressions

You can progress to the single-leg Glute Bridge once the two-legged version has become easy.

Glute Bridge, One Leg

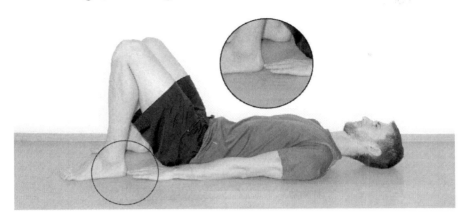

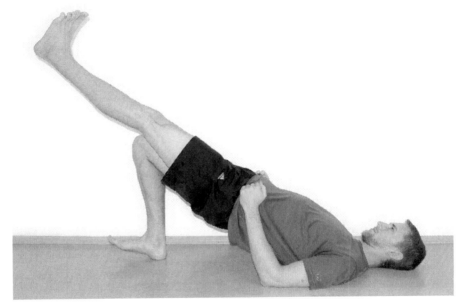

Purpose

The single-leg Glute Bridge improves gluteal activation and strength.

Setup

Lie down on your back and place your arms at your side. Bring your heels back towards your hip so that your fingertips touch your heels.

How to Perform

Lift your toes off the ground so that only your heel is touching the floor. Now lift your hips up as high as you can. Put your hands at the side of your hips to be able to tell if one hip is sagging down. Next, you lift one foot off the ground and extend that leg without losing elevation in your hip. Hold the extended position for the allotted time and then bring the foot back into the starting position. Bring your hips down, relax, and perform the exercise on the other side.

Common Mistakes

- Tensing the hamstrings more than the glutes
- Letting the hip sag
- Letting the hip tilt

Progressions

Once this exercise has become easy you can progress to performing the glute bridge with weight.

Glute Bridge, with Weight

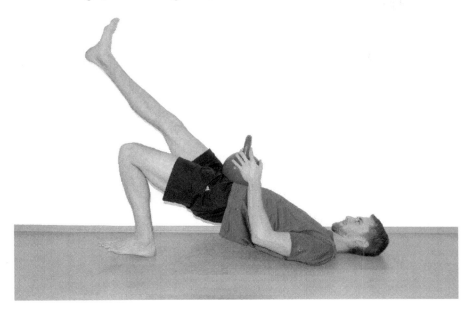

Purpose

Improve the strength of your glutes to increase hip extension force.

Setup

Lie down on your back and place your arms at your side. Bring your heels back towards your hip so that your fingertips touch your heels. Place a weight (*e.g.*, a dumbbell, kettlebell, weight plate, or child) on your lower stomach and make sure it stays put by keeping your hands nearby.

How to Perform

Lift your toes off the ground so that only your heel is touching the floor. Now lift your hips up as high as you can. Put your hands at the side of your hips to be able to tell if one hip is sagging down. Next, you lift one foot off the ground and extend that leg, without losing elevation in your hip. Hold the extended position for a second and bring the foot back into the starting position. Repeat with the other side without letting your hips drop.

Perform the number of repetitions per side without letting your hips come down.

Alternatively, perform all repetitions on one side by extending your hip until you've reached the top position, and then letting your hip drop to the ground again. Next, train the other hip.

Common Mistakes

- Tensing the hamstrings more than the glutes
- Letting the hip sag
- Letting the hip tilt

Regression

Perform the exercise without weight.

Progression

Perform hip thrusts with a barbell (exercise not included).

One-legged RDL, Assisted

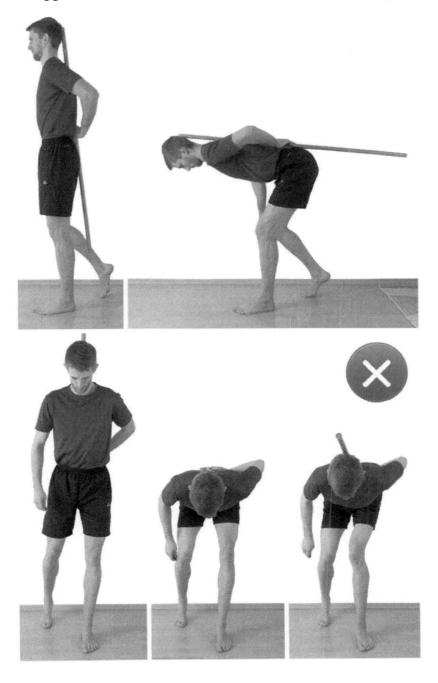

Purpose

Performing the one-legged RDL with a stick helps you figure out proper back alignment. It's an excellent learning aid to discover the technique without using a mirror or filming yourself. The benefits of this exercise go far beyond knee health, as you'll also prevent back pain by learning how to hinge at the hip.

Setup

Stand with your feet slightly less than hip-width apart and your feet pointing forward. Put one foot behind you, with only the toes on the ground. Place the stick behind your back and have it touch your back at the tailbone, the shoulders, and the head.

Make sure the curve behind your lower back isn't too big. I like to hold the stick with two fingers in my lower back area. The lower back has to touch the fingers gently. The pressure should not increase, but your back shouldn't lose contact with the fingers either.

How to Perform

Slightly bend the knee of the working leg and fold your body at the hip. Sit back as you fold your body and only start bending the knee further once your flexibility requires you to.

Maintain proper spinal alignment throughout the movement and reverse it as soon as you start to lose this. Your alignment is off when you lose contact with the stick at your head, shoulders, or tailbone. Your alignment is also off when the curve in your lower back increases or when the pressure your lower back exerts on your fingers increases.

To return to the starting position, you use your glutes and initiate the movement from the hip (i.e., the hip moves first and the knee only "reacts" to this movement).

Your range of motion in this exercise will increase with practice, so don't worry if you cannot touch the ground, as this is not necessary for the exercise to be effective.

Common Mistakes

- Letting the knee travel forward
- Letting the knee collapse inward (see the arrow in the picture)
- Using momentum or bouncing (move in a slow and controlled fashion)

Progressions

Perform this exercise with the other foot not touching the ground ("One-legged RDL, Bodyweight"). This exercise will help you transition to the regular one-legged deadlift.

One-legged RDL, Bodyweight

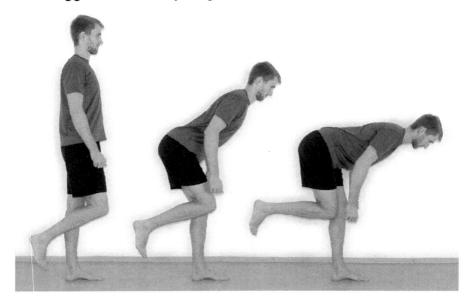

Purpose

The one-legged Romanian Deadlift (RDL) will teach you how to move from the hip, strengthen the muscles on the back of your thigh, and help you to improve your balance. It is also an excellent drill to practice maintaining spinal alignment while bending at the hip.

Setup

Stand with your feet slightly less than hip-width apart and pointing forward. Lift one leg off the floor by bending it at the knee.

How to Perform

Slightly bend the knee of the working leg and fold your body at the hip. Sit back as you fold your body and only start bending the knee further once your flexibility requires you to. Maintain proper spinal alignment (perform the assisted one-legged RDL to learn this) throughout the movement and reverse it as soon as you start to lose this. To return to the starting position, you use your glutes and initiate the movement from the hip (*i.e.,* the hip moves first and the knee only "reacts" to this movement).

Your range of motion in this exercise will increase with practice, so don't worry if you cannot touch the ground, as this is not necessary for the exercise to be effective.

Common Mistakes

- Letting the knee travel forward
- Letting the knee collapse inward
- Using momentum or bouncing (move in a slow and controlled fashion)

Regressions

Perform the assisted one-legged RDL if you haven't done this movement before.

Progressions

Perform the one-legged RDL with loading for an additional challenge. If you don't have access to weights or simply want to stick with the bodyweight variation for a while longer, you can hold the bottom position for a few seconds to stretch your hamstrings under load.

One-legged RDL, with Weight

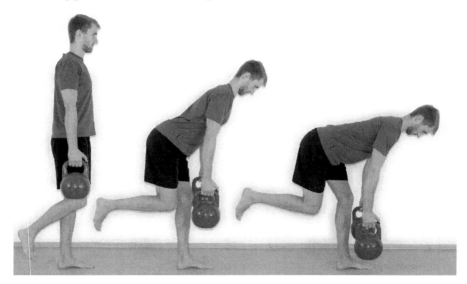

Purpose

The one-legged Romanian Deadlift (RDL) with symmetrical loading allows you to overload the muscles on the back of your leg without the weight pulling your body out of alignment.

Setup

Stand with your feet slightly less than hip-width apart and pointing forward. Hold weights such as kettlebells, dumbbells, or barbell plates in both hands. Lift one leg off the floor by bending it at the knee.

How to Perform

Slightly bend the knee of the working leg and fold your body at the hip. Sit back as you fold your body and only start bending the knee further once your flexibility requires you to. Maintain proper spinal alignment throughout the movement and reverse it as soon as you start to lose this. To return to the starting position you use your glutes and initiate the movement from the hip (*i.e.,* the hip moves first and the knee only "reacts" to this movement).

As with the regular one-legged RDL, it is not necessary to touch the weights to the ground. Perform the exercise in the range of motion in which you can maintain good technique and with time you will be able to go deeper.

Common Mistakes

- Letting the knee travel forward
- Letting the knee collapse inward
- Using momentum or bouncing (move in a slow and controlled fashion)

Regressions

Perform the bodyweight one-legged RDL if you haven't done this movement before.

Progressions

You can use more weight to further increase the challenge of this exercise. You can also hold a weight in one hand and a heavier weight in the hand opposite of the working leg to put asymmetrical loading on your body. With asymmetrical loading you'll have to work harder to maintain alignment.

Two-Legged Jumps

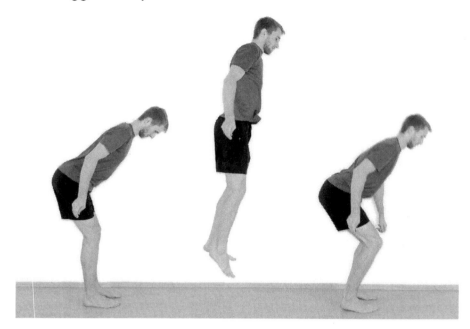

Purpose

Improve basic force absorption technique.

Setup

Stand with your feet hip-width apart.

How to Perform

Fold at the hip like in the one-legged RDL, only with both legs, but bend your knees more. You still have to sit back and most of your weight has to be on your heels. Reverse the movement explosively and press off with the balls of your feet to jump off the ground.

Upon landing, you reverse the movement. The first point of contact are the balls of your feet and you start absorbing the force with your calve muscles. Bring your heels to the ground as silently as possible (think ninja) and once your heels are on the ground you fold back at the hip again. Only flex your knees once you have started bending at the hip (knee flexion occurs secondary to hip flexion). Stand up straight and prepare for another repetition.

Please note that all noise that occurs is the direct result of your body not absorbing the force efficiently. The louder you land, the higher your chances for injury and the worse your technique.

Common Mistakes

- Making a lot of noise (be as silent as possible)
- Letting the knees come forward too much (keep the forward knee movement as small as possible)
- Holding your breath
- Losing proper alignment (*e.g.*, spinal alignment or knees caving in)

Regressions

The goal of this drill is not to increase your explosiveness, but to teach proper jumping technique. For this reason, you only jump as high as you can while maintaining good technique and there is no need to regress this exercise.

Progressions

Perform this exercise on one leg for an additional challenge.

Chapter 6: The Jumper's Knee Treatment Program

This chapter explains the jumper's knee treatment program and its individual training phases. You can download a print-ready version of this plan by going to the online resources page: http://www.fix-knee-pain.com/jumpers-knee-book-guide

Your New Responsibilities

Before we get to the program, I need to remind you that it's your responsibility to discover and do what's right for you. I've created this program to the best of my knowledge, but since there are no one-size-fits-all solutions, you will probably have to adapt it in one way or another.

Additionally, I don't know your individual situation, so if some health issue prevents you from doing certain exercises or if an exercise or stretch doesn't feel right to you, you need to adapt it in a way that makes it possible for you to do that exercise. Adjust your position a bit or use less weight. Scale the exercise to your individual ability.

I've included easier variations of each exercise ("regressions") and it's absolutely no shame to start with easier exercises. Actually, that's what you're supposed to do. Remember, you're not going for records and you're not trying to prove anything by starting with the difficult exercises.

To get the most benefit out of these exercises you need to maintain good technique. Think of it as movement practice, not as working out.

Practice in front of a mirror every now and then to make sure you have good technique and alignment. However, don't make a habit out of practicing in front of a mirror. You want to develop the right body awareness to maintain good technique without visual feedback. After all, once you're performing in your sport there's no one there to hold a mirror for you either.

Training Phase 1: Laying a Strong Foundation

The main goals of the first phase are to improve tissue quality, ankle mobility and hip mobility as well as motor control. We want to ingrain great movement control for the muscles of your hip, which is why you will perform the respective exercises every day. Remember that being able to use those hip muscles is critically important if you want your patellar tendon to stay healthy.

You will do a lot of stretching and mobility work. Additionally, you'll ease into doing the eccentric squats to start strengthening your tendon. Remember: you only need to do the eccentric exercises if you are in the chronic stage of patellar tendonitis. However, if your pain doesn't change with rest, see whether doing the eccentric exercises decreases it.

Daily Exercises

Self-Massage Exercises:

- Adductors
- Calves
- Foot, Underside
- Gluteus Maximus
- Gluteus Medius
- Hamstrings
- IT Band
- Quadriceps: Rectus Femoris
- Quadriceps: Vastus Lateralis
- Quadriceps: Vastus Medialis
- Tensor Fascia Latae

Stretching (for best results, stretch at least twice per day and do each stretch for a total time of at least two minutes per side):

- Hip Flexor Stretch
- Quadriceps Stretch
- Hamstring Stretch
- Calf Stretch

Joint Mobility Exercises:

- Heel Circles, 30 rotations in each direction
- Dorsiflexion Drill, 20 repetitions (do both feet and compare range of motion!)
- Stepping over the fence, 10 repetitions in each direction
- Z-Sit, 15 repetitions in each direction

Strengthening Exercises (increase the number of repetitions slowly from session to session):

- Abduction Drill, 3 sets of 10 to 15 repetitions
- Clams, 3 sets of 10 to 15 repetitions
- Glute Bridge, two-legged, 3 sets of 10 to 15 repetitions
- One-legged RDL, assisted (with Stick), 3 sets of 7 to 15 repetitions

3 to 4 Times per Week: Eccentric Exercises

Based on the studies I came across while doing the research for this book, I think that it's not necessary to do the eccentric exercises every day, like prescribed by the classical jumper's knee treatment.

Collagen synthesis reaches a net positive value 36 hours after exercise (Magnusson et al. 2010), which may be why one researcher had great success with having his clients only do exercises three times per week (Kongsgaard et al. 2009).

However, you still have to do some experimentation to find out what works best for you. Use your training journal and your pain scores to determine which exercise frequency is most effective at reducing your pain. Remember that pain will likely be present during and immediately after exercise, but it should become less in the 24 hours after training.

If your pain stays higher than baseline for more than 24 hours after your training, you've progressed too quickly or made some other mistake.

When you first start out, you can use the general recommendations below and then optimize from there.

Three to four times per week, do the eccentric squats on a slanted board. Start with the two-legged variation and do 3 sets of 10 repetitions. Work your way up to at least 5 sets of 15 repetitions.

Remember to **move slowly** and only increase the repetitions if your pain scores keep falling from week to week!

Phase 1 Bonus Tip

Throughout your day, become aware of movements that stress your patellar tendon and think about ways with which you can relieve some of that stress. For example, when climbing or descending stairs, you can move with a lot of bounce and momentum or you can try to glide up down the stairs gently.

In essence, climbing stairs is like performing many small single-leg squats, either just focusing on the concentric part (when going upstairs) or the eccentric part (when going downstairs). Moving in a controlled fashion is much better for your knees than letting your body sag down the stairs. If you find that going downstairs is too tough for you, you can place more weight on the handrails.

Additionally, pay attention to the alignment of your feet and knees. Do your feet point forward or to the outside? Do your knees cave inward on each step or do they keep tracking properly?

Phase 1 Progression Test

The progression tests are meant to help you determine whether you're ready to go to the next stage of the program. Ultimately, however, your pain scores will tell you whether you were ready to progress or not. If you switch to the next phase and your pain scores stop declining or go up from week to week, you weren't ready yet.

If you've done the phase one training for at least 3 weeks, you can try the progression test. To do the test, perform 3 sets of 15 repetitions of the two-legged eccentric squats on the slanted board. Take at least 3 seconds on the way down and get up the way you've practiced.

Are you mostly pain-free (pain score of 3 or lower)? If so, progress to the second phase of the program.

Training Phase 2: Healing the Tendon

Now that you've rewired your nervous system to be able to use your hip muscles again, we will start to strengthen them with more demanding exercises. Additionally, you will do a tougher variation of the eccentric squats to help your patellar tendons heal further.

Daily Exercises

Stretching (for best results, stretch at least twice per day and do each stretch for at least two minutes per side):

- Hip Flexor Stretch
- Quadriceps Stretch
- Hamstring Stretch
- Calf Stretch

Joint Mobility Exercises:

- Heel Circles, 40 rotations in each direction (achieve as much range of motion as possible)
- Dorsiflexion Drill, 20 repetitions
- Stepping over the fence, 15 repetitions in each direction
- Z-Sit, 25 repetitions in each direction

Every other day or as needed

By now, your tissue quality has improved to a point at which you don't need to perform self-massage every day. Do the self-massage exercises every other day or do them whenever you feel you need to.

Self-Massage Exercises:

- Adductors
- Calves
- Foot, Underside
- Gluteus Maximus
- Gluteus Medius
- Hamstrings
- IT Band

- Quadriceps: Rectus Femoris
- Quadriceps: Vastus Lateralis
- Quadriceps: Vastus Medialis
- Tensor Fascia Latae

3 Times per Week: Strengthening Exercises and Eccentrics

Since the eccentric exercises on one leg demand more balance, you should do them before performing the strengthening exercises.

Strengthening Exercises:

- One-legged RDL, bodyweight, 4 sets of 7 to 15 repetitions
- Abduction Drill with Band, 3 sets of 10 to 15 repetitions
- Clams with Band, 3 sets of 10 to 15 repetitions
- Glute Bridge, one-legged, 3 sets of 10 to 15 repetitions

Eccentric Exercises:

In this phase, you slowly transition from doing two-legged eccentric squats on the slanted board to doing one-legged eccentric squats on the slanted board. Remember to take at least 3 seconds on the way down. The slow movement helps you heal your patellar tendon and is very beneficial for storing good movement patterns.

When you're doing the squats, pay attention to your knee and don't let it cave inwards or move forward out over your toes. The shin of the working leg needs to stay close to vertical.

Some people say only to work the leg with the injured knee, but I prefer to work both legs with equal volume. This prevents muscular imbalances between sides and helps you ingrain good movement control on the non-injured side as well. After all, you're also strengthening the healthy knee by going through these exercises.

In the first week, begin by placing around 75% of your weight on one leg on the way down (the other leg still carries 25%). Use both legs equally to stand up. In the next week, place a little more weight on your working leg (e.g., 85%). Use this method to increase the weight on your working leg from week to week. In time, you will eventually be able to do one-legged eccentric squats to parallel.

Work up to doing 3 sets of 15 repetitions. If you can't maintain a 3-second descent, assist yourself more with the other leg or stop the session. Going slowly is of utmost importance to heal your tendon. If you don't have the strength to maintain good movement technique, you're at great risk of aggravating your injury again.

Remember to pay attention to your pain scores. If your pain scores stay elevated for more than 24 hours after your training, you've progressed too quickly. In that case, decrease your repetition numbers until find a training volume that lowers your pain.

Phase 2 Bonus Tip

In phase 1, you've learned how to use your gluteals, the big strong buttocks muscles. While in phase two, you can actively tense your glutes throughout your day to learn how you can integrate them into a variety of movements. For example, when climbing stairs you can tense your glutes when you reach full hip extension at the end of each step. You can also experiment with tensing your glutes while walking (tense the glute of the rear leg when reaching full hip extension).

This will help teach your motor control center how to activate these muscles properly.

Phase 2 Progression Test

If you've been in this phase for at least 8 weeks, you can try the progression test. Perform 3 sets of 15 repetitions, of the one-legged eccentric squat to parallel. Do it for both legs.

Were you able to do it with almost no pain (pain score of 2 or lower) while maintaining good movement technique (no flailing, losing balance, knees caving inward etc.)? If so, progress to third phase of the program.

Training Phase 3: Getting Your Knees to 100%

Once you're in this phase you will be tempted to return to sports because your knees are almost pain-free. Don't make that mistake! Take at least another month to make sure your tendon is strong enough for the demands of your sport.

In this phase, you will do even more demanding exercises to ensure your movement technique stays good under load.

Daily Exercises

Stretching:

- Hip Flexor Stretch
- Quadriceps Stretch
- Hamstring Stretch
- Calf Stretch

Joint Mobility Exercises:

- Heel Circles, 50 rotations in each direction
- Dorsiflexion Drill, 20 repetitions
- Stepping over the fence, 15 repetitions in each direction
- Z-Sit, 25 repetitions in each direction

Every Other Day or As Needed

Like in phase two, you only need to do the self-massage exercises every other day, or as needed.

Self-Massage Exercises:

- Adductors
- Calves
- Foot, Underside
- Gluteus Maximus
- Gluteus Medius
- Hamstrings
- IT Band

- Quadriceps: Rectus Femoris
- Quadriceps: Vastus Lateralis
- Quadriceps: Vastus Medialis
- Tensor Fascia Latae

2 or 3 Times per Week: Strengthening Exercises and Eccentrics

Like in phase two, do the eccentric exercises before the strengthening exercises. Doing the strengthening drills first would make maintaining balance much harder.

Strengthening Exercises:

- One-legged RDL, with weight, 4 sets of 7 to 12 repetitions (use one or two dumbbells, as heavy as you can safely handle with good technique).
- Abduction Drill with Band, 2 sets of 15 to 20 repetitions
- Clams with Band, 2 sets of 15 to 20 repetitions
- Glute Bridge, one-legged with weight, 3 sets of 10 to 15 repetitions (use however much weight you can safely handle)

Eccentric Exercises:

In this phase, you will transition from just doing the eccentric of the single-leg squat on the slanted board to doing the eccentric and the concentric (to parallel). As before, take at least 3 seconds for the way down. Once you're at parallel, pause for a second, and return to the starting position taking another 3 seconds on the way up.

As I've mentioned before, doing the exercise so slowly is very important to prevent energy storage in your tendon. Additionally, the slow movement will make it impossible to cheat by using momentum.

Moving slowly will ruthlessly reveal any movement problems you still have. Put in extra effort to eradicate all technique problems you uncover (e.g., collapsing knees, feet turning out etc.). The technique you program into your nervous system with this practice will later be called upon when you're performing in your sport, so take your time and do it right.

Start with 3 sets of 6 to 9 repetitions and work your way up to 3 sets of 15 repetitions.

Phase 3 Bonus Tip

If you want to try an advanced joint mobility regimen instead of the same old routine, check out the advanced joint mobility video on the online resources page: http://www.fix-knee-pain.com/jumpers-knee-book-guide/

You will find Coach Scott Sonnon's excellent 30-minute joint mobility routine that he offers free of charge.

This is a valuable resource that will help you uncover hidden joint restrictions in your whole body, remove even more muscle tension, and will make you feel years younger.

Phase 3 Progression Test

Once you can do the slow single-leg squat to parallel for 3 sets of 15 repetitions while being pain-free (pain score of 1 or 2) you have successfully completed the third phase.

To progress further, you can take a backpack and slowly start adding weight to it. Start with 1 pound for the first week and then try two pounds in the week that follows. Alternatively, you can start to transition back into your sport. Either way, remember to keep monitoring your pain scores and to modify your activity level accordingly.

Chapter 7: Preventing Patellar Tendonitis in the Future

In this chapter, you will learn a number of strategies with which you will be able to prevent patellar tendonitis from returning in the future.

1) Don't Overdo It and Use Gradual Increases

The easiest and most obvious way to prevent overuse injuries is to stop overuse. I've already talked about the enthusiasm of athletes in an earlier chapter, so let's focus on how you can achieve a gradual improvement instead.

Regardless of what sport you're performing, you should always use a training journal. The main purpose of the training journal is to provide a record of all the training sessions you did, but you can also make notes about small aches and pains.

Once you've found a training level that you can sustain without pain in your knees, you should maintain that level for a month. Don't worry about the training effect and the need to increase. Even if you lift the same weights for 4 weeks, you'll still derive a training benefit.

After this period, increase only one variable of your training by 10% each week. If you want to increase weight, keep your repetitions, tempo, and rest periods the same. If you want to increase your repetitions, keep the weight, the tempo, and the rest periods the same. This practice ensures that your body "knows" what to adapt to (to learn more about this, check out the book "The Poliquin Principles").

These gradual increases allow your tendons enough time to adapt to the new training load and will prevent overuse.

Additionally, leave two or three days of rest between training sessions that included intense ballistic activities. Going back to the earlier example of the weekend tournament, take Monday, Tuesday, and maybe even Wednesday off if you went through demanding ballistic activities on the weekend. Depending on how you feel, scale the activity on Thursday down to make sure your tendons are safe.

I know this recommendation sounds like a boring approach to fitness, but in the end the race towards becoming a better athlete isn't a sprint, it's a marathon. You're not going to break records by pushing your body to its limits for a couple of weeks (the sprint approach). This approach yield some short-term gains, but at grave long-term costs in the form of injuries.

Only when you stay healthy and motivated for training for years will you be able to achieve serious accomplishments in your sport (the marathon approach).

2) Continue Doing Strengthening Exercises

The slow squats are a safe and easy way to overload your patellar tendons and to stimulate them to grow stronger. You don't need to do keep doing the exercises on the slanted board. Instead, train the single-leg squats to parallel on even ground, holding on some weight.

This is an ongoing process and you won't get from having patellar tendonitis to being able to do single-leg squats with 20 pounds of additional weight in just a few weeks. This kind of strengthening takes many months and requires a lot of persistence on your part, but in the end, it's worth it.

Your legs will be much stronger, your movement control will be better, and your tendons will be healthy.

3) Maintain Strong Supporting Musculature

The same goes for your "supporting" musculature. Your glutes and hamstrings for example. Keep working on gluteal and hamstring exercises and you will improve your athletic potential, while also making sure your knees stay healthy.

Once you've worked through all the glute exercises in this book you can look into advanced exercises for your glutes such as barbell hip thrusts or heavy kettlebell swings.

4) Spend At Least 5 Minutes Every Day on Ankle and Hip Mobility

I know mobility training is somewhat boring, but it's unavoidable if you want to keep improving in your sport. The easiest way to make sure you keep doing it is by plugging it into your daily routine.

Once you've made it a habit, accept no excuses to skip your mobility practice. If you're sick, you'll still do it, maybe a bit more slowly. If you're travelling, you may have to adapt your routine for lack of equipment, but you can still do it.

The payoff is huge.

5) Spend at least 10 Minutes Every Day Stretching

If you have desk job and you know that you don't get enough movement every day, make sure you do at least ten minutes of stretching each day to offset the negative effects long periods spent sitting. Most importantly, stretch your quads and hip flexors.

If you need to, spend some time stretching your calves, and hamstrings.

Alternatively, take on Scott Sonnon's IntuFlow routine (check out online resources page).

6) Keep Practicing Good Movement Quality

Once you've learned what to pay attention to when moving in terms of ankle, knee, and hip alignment, make sure you keep practicing it throughout your day. Watch whether your knees collapse when you're taking stairs, pay attention to where the pressure is underneath your foot when you're walking, investigate any problems that you encounter and experiment to find solutions.

This movement practice also extends into your sport. For example, if you're playing a sport that requires a lot of jumping, do force absorption work. You don't want your tendons to absorb the impact of a landing. Train your muscles to do that. Barefoot training is very valuable to tech proper technique quickly.

Another technique you can use is to record yourself moving and then play it in slow motion. Using a playback program like VLC (http://www.videolan.org/vlc/) you can easily adjust the playback speed by pressing the minus or the plus key (also makes for great entertainment if you have children).

I also highly recommend you go to seminars about your particular sport. If you're into swimming, check out Total Immersion courses. If you're a runner, go to a Pose Running seminar. If you like weightlifting, go to one of Kelly Starrett's seminars. If you're into bodyweight training, check out Steve Maxwell's seminars.

These are excellent resources to take your training to the next level and while some of you may be deterred by the cost of these seminars, let me assure you that it's worth every penny! You'll go home with new ideas, fixed problems, more motivation, new friends, and a big smile on your face.

7) Stop Playing When You Get Fatigued

This goes hand in hand with points 1 and 6. Don't try to improve your athletic capacity on the court. The competitive nature will quickly erode your will to maintain good movement quality. You'll start pushing yourself further, when deep down you know that you should quit while you're ahead.

I've played many basketball games that I shouldn't have played because I was fatigued. Luckily, I wasn't injured. Yet, I'm completely convinced that these extra 20 or 30 minutes didn't give me anything. It wasn't fun, because I was already tired. I didn't improve my game, because my explosiveness was already diminished. All it did was store bad movement patterns in my central nervous system. It's just not worth it.

If you want to push yourself hard, do it during training and with an exercise that will not overstress your tendons. Don't do box jumps for a personal record in repetitions. Instead, do joint-friendly exercises like the kettlebell swing or crawling. Don't believe how tough crawling can be? Look up the spiderman crawl and do it for 20 seconds. Then get back to me:

https://www.facebook.com/photo.php?v=534111429987906

During training, you can fully control all variables of your effort and aren't tempted to prove something. It's a very safe environment to test your boundaries.

8) Cross Train

Take on another sport that uses your body in a different way. If you mostly do endurance activities, do more strength training. Simple bodyweight exercises are enough; you don't need to join a gym. If you're into heavy weightlifting, try something more relaxing like swimming or hiking.

You should also expand your movement horizon in ways that go beyond traditional sports. Check out Ido Portals locomotion video for an excellent demonstration on what variety of movement looks like if it's combined with high movement quality:

https://www.youtube.com/watch?v=G6BBk3Nvj9k

Remember that all specialization comes at a high price. If you specialize in a particular sport, chances are high that you're neglecting many parts of your body and overstressing others. Many excellent triathletes are unable to do one single pull-up for example. Conversely, many very strong individuals can't run a mile without gassing out.

Some may consider this an overly philosophical approach, but are you really a good athlete if your ability is only limited to your specific sport? If you're an excellent runner but can't pull yourself up and over a ledge, is your fitness really that great?

9) Remove Inflammatory Poisons From Your Diet

I've already written about this in detail in my book *Total Knee Health*. In short, there are many inflammatory poisons in our food these days. The worst offenders are vegetable oils (e.g., corn oil, canola oil, safflower oil, soybean oil, and grape seed oil), trans-fats, and sugar.

Avoid these poisons if your life depended on it (because it does).

Supplement with liquid fish oil to make sure your body gets rid those bad fats (more on that in the next chapter).

10) Warm Up Properly

Always warm up properly before games or your training. I like to do a short joint mobility routine that targets the joints that involved in the movements I'm going to practice. Spend at least five to ten minutes warming up to make sure your body is ready for movement. If you feel any tension in parts of your body, use joint mobility and foam rolling to get rid of it.

Additionally, if you play a sport that requires a lot of leg movement, do a short gluteal activation routine. One set of glute bridges, clamshells, and hip abductions will suffice. If you can, throw some band walks in as well. The goal isn't to tire the muscles. You're merely trying to help your nervous system remember how to use these muscles. It may seem like a small thing to do, but the payoff is surprising.

Chapter 8: Dietary Supplements for Patellar Tendonitis

The right dietary supplements can support your recovery from jumper's knee. However, while taking the right supplements can speed your healing, you still have to invest time into finding and fixing the cause for your overloaded patellar tendon. Don't expect your pain to disappear solely because of these supplements, but be proactive about your injury and follow the advice in the previous chapters.

While the supplements mentioned below have helped people with tendonitis, you should bear in mind that these user testimonials present only anecdotal evidence. Little actual research has been done into the efficacy of these supplements for patellar tendonitis and while person A may derive great benefits from taking a certain supplement, the exact same supplement might provide no noticeable benefit for person B.

Lastly, make sure you take the supplement for at least a month before passing judgment. You should consult your physician before starting self-treatment with these supplements.

Fish Oil and Vitamin C

Renowned gymnastics coach Christopher Sommer suggests the use of vitamin C and fish oil to treat tendonitis (Sommer). This makes sense as vitamin C has been shown to improve collagen synthesis (Russell, Manske 1991), while lack of vitamin C, (which causes scurvy) , is associated with decreased collagen synthesis (Grosso et al. 2013; Kipp et al. 1996). High dose vitamin C supplementation has also been shown to enhance tendon healing in studies on rats (Omeroğlu et al. 2009) and is being used in pharmaceutical products that promise to improve tendon healing (Shakibaei et al. 2011).

Coach Christopher Sommer recommends taking one to two grams of vitamin C per day when dealing with tendinopathy (Sommer).

Remember that your body gets used to the amount of vitamin C you ingest and will decrease the absorption. For that reason, it's a good idea to vary the daily intake from day to day. Maintaining an overly high supplementation of vitamin C for a longer time is not advised (you can learn more about the reasons on the online resources page if you want). Hence, only use vitamin C for the initial 8-week period. Taper your vitamin C dose off slowly over a few weeks to allow your body to adapt to lower dietary levels of vitamin C.

Fish oil, on the other hand, has already been proven to have a myriad of health benefits beyond that of improving joint health:

- Helps reduce stress by lowering the amount of stress hormones secreted
- Lowers VLDL cholesterol and triglycerides
- Increases HDL cholesterol
- Improves cognitive abilities (i.e., you'll be smarter)
- Helps you lower your body fat by turning on fat-burning genes
- Will help you build muscle

For more information see (Carter et al. 2013), (Delarue et al. 2003), (Guebre-Egziabher et al. 2013), (Hellhammer et al. 2012), (Poliquin), and (Sofi et al. 2013).

Research into the effects of fish oil supplementation on the treatment of tendinopathy has also revealed positive results (Lewis, Sandford 2009). Additionally, fish oil helps with fixing systemic risk factors for tendonitis. Such risk factors include insulin resistance and excess body fat.

In summary, high-level athletes and coaches utilize fish oil to beat tendinopathy and research has found a beneficial effect as well. Hence, the evidence supporting supplementation with fish oil is strong.

Dosage recommendations for fish oil vary widely. Sought-after Olympic strength coach Charles Poliquin recommends dosages as high as 30 to 45 grams of fish oil per day (Poliquin 2006), which would equal around three tablespoons of liquid fish oil. Ido Portal, a world-class movement teacher, recommends one gram of fish oil per percentage of body fat (Portal). Lastly, Coach Christopher Sommer suggests around two teaspoons per day (Sommer).

The liquid fish oil products I have used give a daily-recommended dose of one teaspoon per day, which seems low compared with what the above-mentioned experts suggest for their clients. A study done on the effects of fish oil supplementation on arthritis joint pain used 2.2 gram of EPA/DHA in the first five weeks and 1.1 gram thereafter (Caturla et al. 2011). This would equal two teaspoons per day or one tablespoon per day, respectively.

I personally take one tablespoon per day and that equals around 2 to three teaspoons, depending on how big the spoon is. Taking around two teaspoons of fish oil is sufficient to derive its benefits.

Fish oil has a blood-thinning effect. Consult your physician before taking this supplement if you're taking any other blood-thinning medication.

Make sure you're getting a pharmaceutical-grade fish oil supplement. In the past, cheaper products have been discovered to contain PCBs and other harmful substances, so do yourself a favor and save money elsewhere or don't buy supplements altogether. Nordic Naturals®, Carlson Labs®, and Pure Encapsulations® are good brands to buy.

Additionally, a liquid fish oil supplement will make it easier for you to get the required dosages of omega-3 fatty acids. Soft gel supplements would require you to take dozens of pills per day to reach the required dosage, which is why they wouldn't last long and be more expensive in the end.

For more information on fish oil and on how you can avoid poisonous dietary fats, go here:

http://www.fix-knee-pain.com/resources/fish-oil/

Cissus

In India, Cissus quadrangularis has been used for medicinal purposes for thousands of years. In recent years, it has also been gaining popularity in the Western world. Studies done on Cissus have mostly concentrated on its bone healing properties. The supplement has been found to speed up the healing of fractures by around 30%, but it's also beneficial for weight loss and has anti-inflammatory properties (Stohs, Ray 2012).

Using the anecdotal evidence offered by online product reviews it becomes clear that while some people with tendinopathy have great results, others didn't notice any improvement at all. About half the people with tendon issues reported improvements, while supplementation didn't show any benefits for the other half. Interestingly enough, Cissus contains vitamin C (Jainu, Devi 2005), which might be why some people with tendonitis noticed an improvement.

Of course, online reviews don't provide definitive proof one way or another, but they do deliver valuable information on how many people had success using a certain supplement for a specific health condition. Using this information in conjunction with research data will help us find the supplements that are most likely to work for treating patellar tendonitis.

Given the research and anecdotal evidence on Cissus, I consider fish oil and vitamin C a more reliable solution when it comes to dealing with tendon issues, especially since more research has been done on the benefits of fish oil and vitamin C. However, if you need to heal a fracture, Cissus should be on your supplement list.

Glucosamine/Chondroitin

When it comes to joint health supplements, glucosamine and chondroitin supplements are usually the first products suggested. Studies have shown these supplements to be beneficial for patients with osteoarthritis (Deal, Moskowitz 1999) and they're generally considered safe for self-supplementation (Vangsness et al. 2009). Glucosamine and chondroitin have also been shown to increase collagen synthesis (Lippiello 2007) and to improve tendon healing in rats (Ozer et al. 2011).

However, taking the anecdotal evidence through online reviews into consideration, the majority of people with tendinopathy didn't notice any benefit from taking glucosamine/chondroitin. The reasons for this lack of efficacy for tendinopathy are unclear. With that being said, fish oil and vitamin C are still a more sound investment into your health.

Move Free © and Other Joint Health Supplements

Move Free© is a joint health compound that contains glucosamine, chondroitin, methylsufonylmethan (MSM), vitamin D, Uniflex© ("fruitex-b calcium fructoborate"), and hyaluronic acid. It can be considered a premium glucosamine/chondroitin supplement and it seems to work well for people with arthritis joint pain.

The added vitamin D is certainly beneficial, since vitamin D deficiencies are common these days, and glucosamine as well as chondroitin have already been established to be useful for people with osteoarthritis.

Research into "fruitex-b calcium fructoborate", has only started a few years ago and while the compound does exhibit anti-inflammatory properties that have been shown to be beneficial for patients with osteoarthritis (Scorei et al. 2011), the actual treatment benefits for tendinopathy are unclear.

The vast majority of online reviews of the various Move Free© products are from people who suffer from osteoarthritis or related conditions. With that being the case and the facts presented in the previous paragraph, I wouldn't recommend this product for tendinopathy. Again, if you have arthritis, give it a shot. Make sure, however, to pay for a liquid fish oil supplement first.

You can evaluate the potential usefulness of the numerous other joint health supplements that are available by looking at their ingredients. If the product contains around 2 grams of the omega-3 fatty acids EPA/DHA and at least one gram of vitamin C you can try it.

However, many brands try to swindle customers by touting omega-3 fatty acids on the cover, but when you look at the ingredient list you'll find that it's only ALA. ALA, alpha-linolenic acid, is an omega-3 fatty acid, but the body is very inefficient at converting it into the important omega-3s EPA and DHA. It's much cheaper though, which is why some companies bolster their margins using ALA from, for example, flaxseed oil. However, these inferior products won't do much for your joints.

To be on the safe side, stick with pharmaceutical grade liquid fish oil and buy a high quality vitamin C supplement.

Natural Anti-Inflammatories

In 2011 and 2012, curcumin was making waves as a newly discovered natural treatment for inflammatory diseases, including tendonitis. The question of whether inflammation is involved with tendonitis is still being discussed and while the majority of researchers now consider tendinopathy void of inflammation, no ultimate consensus has been reached (Rees et al. 2013).

One study has found curcumin to help prevent the breakdown of the extra-cellular matrix and tendon cell death (Buhrmann et al. 2011). Given these findings, curcumin may be beneficial for treating tendinopathy, especially late stage tendinopathy.

Another natural anti-inflammatory that is usually suggested for speeding up recovery after soft-tissue injuries is bromelain. It has been found to improve healing after acute Achilles tendon injuries in rats (Aiyegbusi et al. 2011) and is being used in a number of pharmaceutical products that are geared towards healing soft-tissue injuries. Bromelain also helps with pain.

Don't take Bromelain if you are allergic to pineapple and consult your physician about supplementing with Bromelain if you are taking any blood-thinning medication. Generally, take note of any adverse reactions you experience when supplementing and stop if necessary.

Since no long-term studies exist on the efficacy of supplementing with concentrated doses of these natural anti-inflammatories for treatment of patellar tendinopathy, the safest way to use them is consuming the respective foods. Simply eat more curry and pineapple. While you're at it, add some foods that contain flavonoids, as these are also anti-inflammatory and contain other nutrients that aid in recovery from injury. This includes garlic, cocoa, tea, and blueberries.

You should generally make sure that your diet contains many natural foods and little to no processed foods.

Chapter 9: Other Effective Treatment Options for Patellar Tendonitis

In this chapter, we will briefly look at other treatment options for patellar tendonitis and their effectiveness.

Neurokinetic Therapy™ (NKT)

Neurokinetic Therapy ™ is a relatively new treatment modality and has gained a lot of popularity in recent years for its efficacy in solving chronic pain problems. It works by using muscle testing to identify muscles the brain isn't using properly. This inability to use a muscle properly expresses itself in dysfunctional movement patterns, which will eventually lead to pain in those body parts that are being overloaded to compensate for the weak muscle(s).

NKT then addresses these motor control problems by using muscle testing in combination with exercises that are geared towards resetting the muscle to its normal state, restoring the ability for proper motor control in formerly dysfunctional movement patterns in the process. This allows overloaded muscles that were compensating for the weak muscle to recover. It can also lead to unexpectedly quick recovery from chronic musculoskeletal ailments and other long-standing pain conditions, especially when used in combination with deep tissue laser therapy.

To find a practitioner of NKT in your area, go to http://neurokinetictherapy.com/certified-practitioners

Alternatively, if you are a health care professional and want to learn how you can apply NKT, visit a training seminar. To learn more, go to http://neurokinetictherapy.com/seminars/about

Professional Soft-Tissue Treatment (ART®)

Active Release Technique® is a soft-tissue treatment modality that can help you clear out soft-tissue restrictions. In this treatment modality, the tightness of the tissue is evaluated through the practitioner and the tightness is then released using a number of special massage techniques.

ART® has become very popular among professional and recreational athletes alike. If you know you have soft-tissue problems that you can't solve with the self-massage techniques presented earlier in the book, going to an ART-provider can fix the problem.

To find a provider in your area, go to

http://www.activerelease.com/providerSearch.asp

Two things you have to bear in mind are that ART® can be very uncomfortable and that it does not help you fix dysfunctional movement patterns in the same way that NKT does. Releasing soft-tissue problems goes a long way in restoring healthy movement, but if the movement patterns that are stored in your brain keep you moving in a dysfunctional way, your pain, and the muscle tightness, will reoccur.

In other words, if going to an ART® provider only gives you temporary relief, it's not a good solution for your problem. The same is true for the self-massage exercises presented earlier in this book.

Heavy Slow Resistance Training

In 2009 and 2010, an exciting new treatment protocol for patellar tendonitis was subject of a study by Danish researcher Mads Kongsgaard. Kongsgaard used heavy slow resistance (HSR) training to beat patellar tendonitis (Kongsgaard et al. 2009; Kongsgaard et al. 2010). However, with only two studies supporting HSR, I prefer to go with the tried and true method of eccentric exercises in this book, albeit on an optimized schedule, as eccentric exercises have been proven to work by dozens of studies.

In his research study, Kongsgaard had his participants perform slow weightlifting exercises with heavy resistance, taking 3 seconds for the eccentric and 3 seconds for the concentric part of the movement. The exercises they performed were the back squat, the hack squat, and the leg press.

Let me briefly summarize why I don't recommend his treatment protocol. First, eccentric exercises on a slanted board have been proven effective for patellar tendinopathy in numerous studies over the past 15 years. HSR is certainly an exciting new treatment option, but with only one randomized control study supporting it.

Second, not everyone has access to the required equipment. While most gyms offer a leg press, you won't be able to find a hack squat machine that easily. Finding a gym with a squat rack, which should be used to perform back squats safely, is like hitting the lottery. Finally, if a gym has a squat rack, it's often constantly in use, leaving little time to complete the exercises.

In addition to the equipment required for the exercise, the back squat also requires the trainee to be familiar with the technique of the exercise. Outside of powerlifting circles, most trainees would need the help of a qualified personal trainer to learn the back squat. Even if you know the proper technique, handling heavy loads on your back while squatting slowly puts your back at risk, as the spinal stabilization provided by your core muscles will be under constant tension and eventually fatigue.

I suspect slowly performed single-leg exercises such as the single-leg squat are a viable alternative to the exercises suggested by Kongsgaard, and have tried to contact the author with questions regarding this substitution. However, I've yet to hear back from him.

If you want to try the HSR protocol, go checkout the study at http://www.ncbi.nlm.nih.gov/pubmed/19793213

Therapeutic Ultrasound

Therapeutic ultrasound uses high frequency sound waves that cannot be heard by humans to stimulate the tissue under the skin. In research studies, there is no clear consensus on whether therapeutic ultrasound can work for patellar tendinopathy or not. Some studies say it works (Tsai et al. 2011), while others quote inconsistent results (Andres, Murrell 2008). The majority of researchers found that therapeutic ultrasound provides no benefit when healing tendinopathy (Larsson et al. 2012, p. 1645; Chester et al. 2008; Warden et al. 2008).

One study found that applying Aloe Vera Gel and aiding its penetration into the skin with ultrasound helped improve realignment of collagen (Maia Filho et al. 2010). Then again, it's only one study. When researchers compared eccentric exercises with therapeutic ultrasound, eccentric exercises yielded better results (Stasinopoulos, Stasinopoulos 2004).

With these results in mind, I can't recommend therapeutic ultrasound for tendinopathy.

Extra Corporal Shockwave Therapy

ESWT uses acoustic waves with a very high energy to deliver a mechanical stimulus to the treatment area. ESWT has been shown to be beneficial for treating Achilles tendinopathy (Rowe et al. 2012) and patellar tendinopathy (Furia et al. 2013). Another study found that ESWT could yield results comparable to those of eccentric training (Rompe et al. 2006).

However, in 2012 a systematic review of available studies, the authors concluded that more research into ESWT for patellar tendinopathy needs to be performed before it can be recommended (Larsson et al. 2012, p. 1645).

If your physician wants to perform ESWT on your patellar tendon, make sure he has enough experience in applying it for this condition, as improperly applied ESWT can damage the tendon (Sharma, Maffulli 2008, p. 1739). Your physician should have produced good results in the past.

Laser Treatment

Laser therapy accelerates the healing process of damaged tissue by stimulating the cellular metabolism. To learn more about how laser treatment works, check out the respective video on the online resources page.

Low-level laser treatment has been shown to increase collagen formation (Sharma, Maffulli 2008, p. 1739) and to provide a better long-term outcome for patients with patellar tendinopathy (Sussmilch-

Leitch et al. 2012). However, it's important to remember that these results were obtained with low-power lasers. Lasers that are more powerful can penetrate deeper into the body, thereby leading to better results.

One company that produces these lasers is LiteCure® and their products are already being used by several Major League Baseball teams such as the Boston Red Sox (Starkey). To learn more about this treatment modality and to find a practitioner in your area, go to http://www.litecure.com/

Surgery

Research has found eccentric exercises to provide superior results when compared to surgery (van Usen, Pumberger 2007, p. 8); however, if eccentric training and other treatment modalities have proven unsuccessful, surgery might be the last resort. Unfortunately, surgery provides inconsistent outcomes (Andres, Murrell 2008) and it is unclear how surgically removing damaged issues affects healing, the overall outcome, and pain (Tan, Chan 2008).

If you decide to have surgery, make sure you're in the hands of a surgeon who has experience with patellar tendinopathy.

PRP-Injections

Platelet-rich plasma injections are a minimally invasive procedure in which a substance made from your own blood is injected into your body, in some cases using the guidance of ultrasound to find the exact site of injury in the tendon.

PRP has gained a lot of popularity because numerous professional athletes used it to recover from injuries and several of them made impressive comebacks.

Dr. Michael Hall and colleagues summarize the current research in an article for the New York University Hospital for Joint Diseases as follows: For patellar tendinopathy, PRP injections have been shown to improve pain in patients at a 6 month follow up. In this study, three injections had been used at an interval of 15 days. However, when compared to a historical cohort that was treated conventionally, no statistical differences were found between the PRP-group and the group that received the standard treatment (Hall et al. 2013, p. 57).

Hall et. al conclude that there is little evidence to show an effect greater than placebo and that more studies are needed to confirm the efficacy of PRP-injections (Hall et al. 2013, p. 57).

In another article, Dr. Hall's colleague, Dr. Cardone posits that the beneficial effects of PRP-injections might have occurred because the injection needle damaged the tissue, causing the body to send blood to the area (Cardone). For a good summary about PRP-injections, go to http://www.scientificamerican.com/article.cfm?id=platelet-rich-plasma-therapy-dennis-cardone-sports-medicine-injury (if you don't want to type this long URL, go to http://www.fix-knee-pain.com/jumpers-knee-book-guide/ instead. There are links to relevant articles on this page.)

Conclusion about other Treatment Modalities

If you want to utilize other treatment modalities to aid your recovery from patellar tendinopathy, you should go with non-invasive methods that have been shown to be beneficial first. This list includes Neurokinetic Therapy™, high power laser therapy with class IV lasers, and ART® massages.

If your physician has experience in treating patellar tendinopathy with extra-corporal shockwave therapy, you can also try ESWT.

If non-invasive procedures fail or are not an option, go with a minimally invasive treatment option such as PRP-injections.

Finally, if you've exhausted all other options, your only remaining choice is surgery.

Chapter 10: Frequently Asked Questions

This chapter provides answers to commonly asked questions about patellar tendonitis.

Does patellar tendonitis heal on its own?

If you're in the beginning stages of the injury, reactive tendinopathy or early dysrepair (see chapter two for more information about that), the tendon will repair itself as long as you reduce the load you place on it. Reduce the number of weekly training sessions that stress your knee to one or two sessions and keep them brief. Diligently avoid all exercises that increase your pain. Start supplementing with liquid fish oil and vitamin C to aid the healing process.

If you've progressed to the more serious injury stages, late dysrepair, or degenerative tendinopathy, you need to use the tendon healing exercises discussed in the earlier chapters if you want your pain to decrease. This is because the tendon needs additional stimulation to start the regeneration process again. Rest won't cut it in this case.

Either way, you need to address additional factors that can contribute to patellar tendonitis (see chapter 3).

How do I know when my knees have healed?

During the weeks you perform the treatment exercises, pain levels will slowly decrease. In most research experiments, pain decreased markedly over the course of 12 weeks, by which time some athletes returned to their sport. However, only few were completely pain-free after 12 weeks of doing the rehab exercises. The majority of participants still had low levels of pain or discomfort.

Based on what you've learned in this book, you understand that even being pain-free is not a good indicator for tendon health. However, you can still use pain or discomfort in your knees to determine whether an exercise is safe for you to perform or not. If an exercise increases or causes pain, your tendon is not strong enough or your technique is bad. If you're sure your technique is good, then the activity is still too demanding for your knees.

Increase playing time by only 10% per week and build your volume up gradually over months. If your knees give you any trouble at all, you go back to a level at which they were pain-free and stay there for a few weeks longer before trying to increase playing time again. Pay utmost attention to proper movement technique to minimize the load on your patellar tendon.

The only way to be sure about the health of your knees (other than diagnostic imaging and maybe biopsies) is to continue the rehab exercises for another month or two after your pain has disappeared. After that has happened, you can ease back into your sport, starting with decreased playing time, lowered activity level, and fewer sessions per week.

My knees hurt when doing squats. Should I stop?

This topic is controversial. Some researchers had their participants perform exercises in pain, others preferred to avoid pain as much as possible (Rutland et al. 2010). Depending on how far you've progressed in the injury stages, a certain level of discomfort may be unavoidable.

The important thing is that your pain scores decrease once you've implemented the exercises. Pain should never stay high for more than 24 hours after an exercise. If it does, you put too much stress on your knees during the training.

Make sure you move slowly and scale the exercise down by taking load off your knees if the pain is too severe.

Will running prevent the healing process?

Whether or not a certain exercise prevents the healing process depends on how far your injury has progressed and the quality of your technique for the exercise . Exercise that does not cause pain is usually beneficial for the healing process, as you're increasing blood circulation and are actually using your tendons. In other words, if your running doesn't cause or increase pain, you don't have to worry about it.

However, if you feel slight discomfort in your knees after you've taken a run you know that it was too much. Reduce your running time, train on a softer surface, and take other measures to limit the load you're placing on your knees.

If you're only running to stay in shape, replace it with a low-impact activity such as kettlebell swings, weightlifting, swimming, or biking. When biking, make sure you go for a high cadence to minimize load on your knees. Additionally, have your bike fitted by professional to prevent biking-related overuse injuries from occurring.

Should I use heat or cold?

The common recommendation for patellar tendonitis is to use ice to bring the inflammation down. As you've learned in the earlier chapters, the role of inflammation in patellar tendonitis is still being discussed, with the majority of researchers now agreeing that it's void of inflammation. That calls the practice of icing for tendinopathy into question.

One study done on the long-term effects of icing for lateral elbow tendinopathy found that ice provides no treatment benefit other than a reduction of pain (Manias, Stasinopoulos 2006). This analgesic, or pain-numbing, effect seems to the only benefit icing provides for tendinopathy.

If you have a pain flare-up and don't want to use painkillers, you can ice the area for a couple of minutes until your pain is reduced. However, bear in mind that since icing lowers the pain, you'll have less input to judge whether a certain activity is too stressful for your knees.

When I was dealing with chronic patellar tendinopathy, I actually found heat to be beneficial. Gymnastics Coach Christopher Sommer also recommends trying heat when dealing with tendinopathy (Sommer).

Don't use heat after your training, if you've just sustained an injury, or if you're experiencing patellar tendonitis for the first time. In these cases, icing may help you reduce the pain. If you've had patellar tendonitis pain for more than a couple of weeks you can try heating your knees several times during the day.

To apply heat you can use a warm water bottle, a heating blanket, or a one of these gel packs for icing that you can also heat. Don't burn yourself with too much heat. Leave the heat on for a couple of minutes or until your warm water bottle/gel pack has gotten cold. I recommend you wrap an additional blanket around your knees to help keep the heat in.

You can also apply heat before your training or game to help improve circulation in your joints. Wearing a neoprene sleeve can help keep your knees warm during the game. When playing basketball, I used to wear my old volleyball kneepads, which had the added bonus of protecting my knees against direct trauma.

Granted, I was the only one playing with kneepads, but I was also the only one playing with a mouth guard and the only one properly warming up before games. In my experience, most of the time it's better not to do what everyone else is doing.

Can Jumper's Knee be cured without invasive therapy?

Whether or not a certain treatment modality works for you depends on your individual injury. Generally, results of non-invasive treatment modalities for jumper's knee are very good and you have many options to exhaust before invasive therapy becomes your only choice.

If you haven't been able to get rid of patellar tendonitis, get in touch with a Neurokinetic Therapy practitioner:

http://neurokinetictherapy.com/

What are these crackling noises?

Joint noises can have a number of reasons. Cracking and popping commonly occur because of pressure changes within the joint and the resultant collapse of small bubbles of air. Joint clicking, on the other hand, can occur if you have lax joints or move without good biomechanics.

If these sounds are not accompanied by pain, you shouldn't worry about it. However, if the noises only occurred after an injury or if you feel it's related to your pain, you should consult your doctor about it.

For more information on joint noises, check out the excellent article by Dr. Steven Low I've referenced on the online resources page.

What about patellar tendon straps?

Patellar tendon straps help distribute the load differently inside the tendon by exerting some pressure. Although I haven't found any research about the advantages and disadvantages of patellar tendon straps, I think that they're just a crutch with which you should be very careful. Let me explain.

As you've learned in the book, not all parts of the tendon progress at the same pace throughout the injury stages. Certain parts of the patellar tendon will start to break down first, while others are still healthy. The injured parts had to withstand higher forces during your activity. If you use a tendon strap, the load will be distributed differently throughout the tendon.

Once the load distribution has changed, the pain might decrease. Once the pain decreases, an athlete usually returns to his previous level of play. However, the giant danger here is that this athlete hasn't fixed the underlying cause for the patellar tendon becoming overloaded in the first place. Even in the unlikely event that the injured part of the patellar tendon is able to recover, he or she is still at very great risk of injuring other parts of the tendon as well.

Once more parts of the tendon have been injured, recovery time will be much longer, and that extra month of play the patellar tendon has granted you, will cost you at least an extra month of recovery.

If you need a patellar tendon strap just to be able to go to work and be pain-free throughout the day, it is ok. However, if you use the tendon strap to continue doing sports because you're too lazy to address the actual causes for your pain it will eventually come back and bite you.

Can I use painkillers (e.g., Ibuprofen)?

In her work on tendinopathy, Dr. Jill Cook hypothesizes that the use of NSAIDs such as Ibuprofen or the use of corticosteroids may be beneficial in the very early stages of patellar tendinopathy. However, Cook also warns that both NSAIDs and corticosteroids will slow down tendon repair (Cook, Purdam 2009, p. 413). Other researchers agree about the potential usefulness of NSAIDs and corticosteroids for short-term relief (Andres, Murrell 2008).

If icing isn't enough and you need painkillers to be able to bear the pain, use them for a short time (i.e., not more than a couple of days). Remember that NSAIDs and corticosteroids will weaken your tendon. If you've used either of these substances, you need to take it easy in your training for at least 8 weeks or you risk further tendon injury.

Only use these substances under the guidance of a qualified healthcare professional who knows about their detrimental effects to soft-tissue healing. For example, cortisone increases your risk for tendon rupture. Make sure you avoid all activities that place excessive stress on your tendons to prevent that from happening.

Don't use NSAIDs or corticosteroids when you're trying to recover from chronic cases of patellar tendonitis (i.e., tendinosis), as they will slow down or even prevent soft-tissue healing. A randomized control trial found corticosteroids to provide an unfavorable long-term outcome when compared with eccentric exercises (Kongsgaard et al. 2009). Use ice if you need a way to deal with temporary flare-ups of pain.

Do certain shoes cause patellar tendonitis?

Since standing on a slanted surface increases the load on your patellar tendon, it seems logical that shoes with an elevated heel will place more load on your patellar tendon as you move. Additionally, such shoes will slowly reduce your ankle dorsiflexion, as your ankle doesn't have to bend far if the heel is permanently elevated. That being said, most shoes with an elevated heel will increase your risk for patellar tendonitis to a certain degree and you'd be well advised to stick with flat-soled shoes if you want your feet and ankles to stay healthy.

Moreover, there are certain shoes that claim to support the ankle to prevent ankle sprains. High-top basketball and hiking shoes come to mind. These shoes artificially restrict range of motion at the ankle and while they lower your risk for low ankle sprains, they increase load on your knee. This is because the body will compensate for the restricted ankle range of motion by increasing range motion demands at the knee, slowly leading to overload.

Lastly, if you want to experience the difference shoes make for your movement, just try to play your sport without shoes on. You will go through a relearning process, as your body is unable to exert as much force on the ground without the artificial support of your shoes. Even something as simple as walking on concrete is much different without shoes on and as soon as you remove your shoes, your body will begin to utilize naturally available methods for shock-absorption, which takes time to train and improve.

Barefoot training is an interesting topic that is beyond the scope of this book. If you decide to try it, make sure you do so with light exercises. Increase your training load slowly (10% per week) to make sure you aren't injured. Most people ignore this warning and overdo barefoot training. The consequences are overuse injuries that can be as serious as stress fractures in your foot. Account for these risks properly and barefoot training can be a useful addition to your routine.

Should I rest completely?

If your knees are hurting for the first time then yes, resting completely for two or three days is a good option. See how the pain changes and if rest helps, you can add some additional days.

However, don't rely on rest for more than a week. Inactivity will slowly weaken your tendons, decreasing their tensile strength in the process. Such weakened tendons are at a higher risk of developing tendinopathy in the future.

For this reason, you should perform activities that don't provoke your pain. Any activity that doesn't cause or increase pain helps with the recovery process. However, try to stay away from ballistic exercises and stick to low-impact training for some time so that you give your tendons enough stimuli to heal and stay strong, but don't overload them.

I'm always travelling. How should I train?

If there is no option of training on a slanted surface, you will have to adapt the eccentric exercises to that situation. To do that, you can start by using isometric holds in the first phase. With your back against a wall, get into the squat position, and hold for time.

Once your pain has decreased, you can progress to doing bodyweight squats on even ground. Remember to use your pain scores to gauge whether you're progressing too quickly. Do the bodyweight squats slowly and work towards reclaiming full range of motion.

Once you can do full range body weight squats with a very low level of pain or discomfort, you can start to ease into single-leg squats to parallel. Pay attention to good form and move slowly.

Chapter 11: Your Step-By-Step Treatment Guide

This chapter will summarize the steps you need to take to start healing your patellar tendonitis. If you're reading this on a device that doesn't allow you to click on links, you can go to http://www.fix-knee-pain.com/jumpers-knee-book-guide for a list of referenced resources.

1) Download and print the summary of the training phases

The online resources page offers an overview of the different training phases. Download this overview at the link listed above.

2) Download and keep the exercise technique reminders handy

Online you can also download a file with pictures and a description of each exercise. You can keep this file on your phone or print it. The idea is to make it easier for you to remember the specific exercises.

3) Get a training journal and a slanted board

The resources page also has links to schematics for a slanted board, as well as links where you can buy ready-made models online.

4) Get a RumbleRoller or another foam roller

Get yourself a RumbleRoller or another foam roller. You will need it for the self-massage exercises. As stated earlier, some gyms offer foam rollers, so you might not need to buy one.

5) Get some liquid Fish Oil and Vitamin C

Buy some liquid fish oil and vitamin C. Links to good products are on the online resources page. Alternatively, buy high quality brands such as Nordic Naturals®, Pure Encapsulations®, or Carlson Labs®.

6) Stop all activities that you suspect might have cause or contributed to the pain

Avoid all exercises that increase your pain. If you're playing sports competitively, you will have to weigh the pros and cons of continuing to compete with your injury. What do you stand to gain by keeping playing? Is it worth several extra months of rehab?

7) Start with the first phase of the training program

Start with the first phase of the training program, but leave out the squats for a week or two to establish a good baseline of knee pain and to give your knees some rest. If you've already given your knees rest or if you've had the pain for a longer period of time (several weeks), you can start the full program right away.

8) Write down which exercises you did, how many reps and sets, in your journal

Use your training journal to write down all the exercises you did, how many sets you did, and how many repetitions per set you did.

9) Write down all other activities you did on that day if they have stressed your knees

Did you go for a hiking trip or spent three hours carrying heavy boxes? Write it down in your training journal. This extra activity might cause a flare up in pain that you might otherwise blame on the training program.

10) Write down your pain score throughout the day

Additionally, use your training journal to write down your pain score at a set time each day. For example, write down your pain at noon every day. Make sure you take your pain score before your training.

11) Use your pain scores on the days after a training session to adapt the squats

Experiment with the repetition and set numbers for the eccentric exercises to find a combination that works for you. Each case of patellar tendonitis is different, which is why the rep/set recommendations made in this book are only useful as a starting point from which you need to optimize for your particular situation.

Remember to move slowly when squatting. There should be absolutely no momentum and you can even go as slow as 5 seconds down and 5 seconds up.

12) Once you can pass the progression test for phase one, progress to phase 2

Once you've spent enough time in phase one and feel confident about trying the progression test, give it a shot and see if it affects your pain scores. If you pass the test, move on to phase two. If you don't pass the test, spend some more weeks in phase one and try again later. Remember that rehab is not a race.

13) Get a Theraband or another rubber band you can use for the exercises

For some of the exercises in phase two you will need a Theraband or another rubber band. Buy one online or somewhere else if you don't have one already.

14) Proceed with phase two

Start working on phase two of the training program. Keep using your pain scores to track your progress and adapt the eccentric exercises accordingly.

15) Once you can pass the phase two progression test, progress to phase 3

Once you've spent enough time in phase two and are feeling confident about trying the progression test, give it a try and see if your pain scores change. If you pass the test, move on to phase three. Just like before, if you don't pass the test, spend some more weeks in phase two.

16) Proceed with phase three

Keep tracking your pain scores as you go through the phase three program.

17) Complete the program by passing the phase three test

You've completed the training once you can pass the phase three progression test. If you fail the test, give your knees a few more weeks to get stronger and then try the test again.

18) Follow the advice given in chapter 7 to prevent patellar tendonitis from returning

Once you've completed the training program, follow the advice given to you in chapter 7 to prevent patellar tendonitis from returning in the future. Don't risk several months of work over a small mistake that could have been prevented easily.

Chapter 12: Professional Sports and Patellar Tendonitis

In July of 2013, I had the honor of spending a day with the German National volleyball team when they were preparing for the European Championship. One of their athletic trainers, Alessandro Bracceschi, had invited me to investigate whether the training could be fine-tuned for healthier knees after he had read my book *Total Knee Health* (which he later told me was recommended to him by another professional volleyball player). This chapter covers what I've learned about managing patellar tendonitis in professional sports in the time with the team.

For recreational athletes, the most important piece of advice in this book is to stop ballistic activities when dealing with patellar tendonitis. This will prevent your injury from progressing into the advanced stages and gives you optimal conditions for healing. However, if you're preparing for the European Championship, or if you're being paid to perform at a high level, stopping your training is not an option. So what else can you do?

The first thing you should do is to make sure you use optimal movement technique during strength and skill training. Use the factors mentioned earlier in this book to achieve the lowest possible load on your patellar tendons. This entails aligning your feet to point forward, your knees to keep tracking above your toes (no inward collapse), and to prevent your knees from travelling too far forward out over your knees.

The coach has to monitor alignment during every exercise in the strength-training regimen. This will prevent unnecessary load from being placed on the knees and will help develop good movement habits that will eventually carry-over to the game. If the athlete is unable to correct alignment during a certain exercise, limitations in ankle and hip mobility may be the problem. The exercise can be performed at slower speeds or with lighter weights to allow proper reprogramming of the motor control center.

The demands of the sport may necessitate violating the rules of alignment during certain movements. Working at the net in volleyball prevents the athlete from jumping with a good hip hinge pattern and they therefore have to combine hip hinge with increased knee flexion to maintain an upright torso. In situations like these, the main area in which you can make improvements is the strength training.

Adapting Strength Training to Manage Patellar Tendonitis

In sports that already place a high demand on the knee extensor mechanism, additional knee-dominant work has to be balanced carefully with hip-dominant movements. Knee-dominant movements are movements that place high loads on the knee joint and the muscles on the front of the leg (quadriceps). The torso usually stays upright.

In hip-dominant movements, the hip takes up more of the load and the torso doesn't stay upright. More load is placed on the hamstrings and glutes.

Classic examples of knee-dominant movements are squats and lunges. Good examples of hip-dominant movements are the kettlebell swing, the deadlift, and other movements that primarily work hip extension such as glute bridges or hip thrusts. Granted, certain knee-dominant movements such as the deep squat also load the hips, but it's still a knee-**dominant** exercise.

To keep your knees healthy, maintain a 1:1 ratio between hip- and knee-dominant training.

If an athlete has become symptomatic, the ratio should shift towards more hip-dominant work. In very serious cases, even dropping quad-dominant strength work from the training can be a viable option, since athletes with patellar tendonitis usually already have strong quads and an impressive vertical leap. The quads will get ample stimulus during ball practice, which is why strength as well as explosiveness will mostly be maintained.

In contrast, if you insist on putting the symptomatic athlete through the same training regimen as their healthy teammates, you risk escalating the injury to an advanced stage during which the athlete's performance may then be limited by increased pain. In this scenario, the athlete may have slightly stronger legs, but the pain will prevent the athlete from using them to their full capacity.

With that in mind, spending more training time on hip-dominant work is a more logical choice. It won't lead to more tendon breakdown, can help take load off the knee during sports (as more load is being handled by the glutes and hamstrings), and will aid in keeping the athlete's spirits up since they can still do strength work with their teammates.

Lastly, performing some slow quad-dominant exercises (or isometrics) can be useful to stimulate the collagen fibers to return to good alignment and may help lower the pain.

For best results, the modification of the strength training should be combined with the other treatment modalities mentioned in this book. This can be deep tissue laser treatment, professional soft-tissue treatment, Neurokinetic Therapy, or a combination of these. Supplementing with liquid fish oil is also beneficial.

Current Limitations

Collagen synthesis and tissue turnover occur at a set speed inside the tendon. Without means to change these two factors, the only way to treat patellar tendonitis is to allow for ample rest in between training sessions that stress the patellar tendon. When training through the injury, the athlete may be able to prevent further escalation by intelligently modifying his training as described earlier, but recovery is unlikely during these circumstances.

In other words, the approach presented in this book will work well for recreational athletes, but is insufficient for professional athletes while in season. We are in dire need of more advanced methods of dealing with patellar tendonitis and I intend to search for ways to do that.

To stay up to date with new discoveries, sign up to the patellar tendonitis newsletter on the online resources page:

http://www.fix-knee-pain.com/jumpers-knee-book-guide/

You will also receive a very detailed e-mail course on the most common causes for knee pain. Obviously, I can't make any promises, but I'm highly motivated to dig deeper into this topic and will share my findings with you if you sign on.

Conclusion: Three Paragraph Summary of Jumper's Knee

Jumper's knee is an overuse injury of the patellar tendon. However, whether or not your patellar tendons will be overloaded depends on more than just your training time. Several additional factors, such as ankle range of motion, gluteal strength, and hamstring flexibility, influence how much load your tendons have to handle. Because they can dramatically increase the stress on your patellar tendon, these often-overlooked factors could also be considered hidden causes for patellar tendonitis.

To resolve patellar tendonitis, you have to cease the overuse and fix all factors that contributed to your tendons becoming overloaded. Next, you have to help your tendon grow stronger by using specific exercises for that goal. Additionally, you can use supplements such as fish oil and vitamin C to speed up the healing process. To speed your healing up even further, you can use additional treatment modalities for jumper's knee, such as Neurokinetic Therapy® or professional soft-tissue treatment.

Once you've healed your jumper's knee, you need to abide by several rules to make sure the injury doesn't return in the future. Most importantly, stop activities that cause pain. Find ways to modify your activity so that it doesn't cause pain, like reduced intensity or improved technique (or both). Additionally, you need to keep working on the factors that influence how much load your tendons have to handle. Lastly, keep supplementing with fish oil and clear all inflammatory poisons, such as vegetable oils and processed foods, from your diet.

Bonus Section

The following pages were taken from my book Total Knee Health. I've included these excerpts to provide you with additional information.

Total Knee Health, chapter 3, excerpt:

The 10 Pillars of Knee Health

In a previous chapter, we examined a number of knee pain diseases and you might have already noticed a common theme among them. There actually are several important prerequisites for knee health that when ignored can lead to or exacerbate pain in your knees. The following list will equip you with the basic knowledge that is necessary to start on your path to healthy knees. You should consider all factors to be of equal importance.

Good dietary choices

The connection between diet and knee health is obvious and obscure at the same time. Take weight gain caused by bad dietary choices for example. Any amount of excess body fat places undue load on the joints, which is why overweight people are more likely to suffer from knee and ankle pain. When it comes to body composition, a proper diet is of utmost importance, as shown by the fitness industry mantras "You can't out-train a bad diet" and "Abs are built in the kitchen". The role of exercise during a fat-loss program is merely to minimize muscle tissue breakdown, which would readily occur if one were to diet without exercise.

The connection between diet and joint health goes way beyond body fat percentage though. For example, if you eat too much of the wrong fats your body will enter a low-level state of inflammation. In this state, you're more likely to develop inflammatory diseases. Another important dietary factor is carbohydrate intake. The more you burden your body with carbs in excess of your needs, the more you demineralize your teeth and bones. This puts you at a significantly increased risk for diseases such as tooth decay and osteoporosis.

Additionally, refined carbohydrates will feed the unfriendly bacteria in your gut and make you more likely to develop or extend a yeast or parasite infection. Those kinds of infections are known to alter your immune system and are speculated to be one of the many causes for today's epidemic of autoimmune disorders (*e.g.,* asthma, rheumatoid arthritis, skin disorders).

As you can see, there are more than enough connections between diet and knee health to warrant inclusion of this important aspect of health. Additionally, you can find three very valuable resources that will provide you with the foundational knowledge on diet and nutrition at the end of this book. Everyone looking to improve their health should give those a thorough read. Those not interested in all the details will be provided with everything they need to know about proper dietary choices for joint health in chapter 8.

Strong gluteal muscles

Put simply, the main function of the gluteal muscles is to move your thigh backwards and outwards (hip extension and abduction), but they also enable you to rotate your thigh outwards (external rotation). On top of that, the glutes are relied on to resist movement in the opposite directions. This means if your gluteal muscles are weak you're less able to prevent your thigh from travelling forward or inward. You're also less able to prevent excessive internal rotation.

Initially this may "just" put excessive stress on the front of your knees, leading to diseases such as a degeneration of the patellar or quadriceps tendon, but the long-term risks associated with weak gluteal muscles are more severe. If you have weak or dysfunctional gluteals, your risk of a traumatic knee injury, such as an ACL-tear, increases dramatically, mainly because you're less able to control movement at the hip and your knee is merely slave to what happens at hip and ankle.

Another interesting aspect is that your muscle strength may be good enough to create acceptable movement control, but your nervous system might not know how to use the muscles. This kind of dysfunction can be the result of an injury, but in the vast majority of cases, it is the result of poor movement habits in daily life, like sitting for hours on end every day.

If you sit a lot, your nervous system will adapt the preset for the desired length of your muscles to this posture. The muscles on the backside of your hips are "lengthened", whereas the hip flexors are "shortened", since the hip is in a permanent state of flexion. Those muscles work in antagonistic pairs and if one of them is neurologically shortened, the other becomes inhibited. In the case of sitting a lot, the hip flexors have become short and your gluteals have become inhibited. Over time, your nervous system might even "forget" how to use the gluteal muscles.

For those reasons, it is vital to first reestablish proper motor control of the gluteals and only then strengthen them. This way you ensure their best possible function and good control of thigh movement during jumping, running, cutting and many other athletic movements.

There are several more reasons why strong and healthy gluteal muscles are important. For example, one has to do with the hamstrings becoming overworked if the glutes don't work properly. The hamstrings and glutes normally both contribute to hip extension. If the glutes are weak, the hamstrings have to contract harder to make up for the lost force. In time, this will lead to overworked hamstrings, which have become tight in the process. In very serious cases, this can lead to hamstring tears if the muscle is continually overworked.

In summary, strong and functional gluteals will not only keep you on the playing field by preventing injury, but they will also increase your athletic performance and improve your body composition.

Strong hamstring muscles

The hamstrings are the muscles on the back of your thighs. They contribute to knee flexion, hip extension and hip internal, as well as hip external rotation. The hamstrings also prevent excessive forward movement of the shinbone, thereby acting as an active knee stabilizer. This means your hamstrings and your ACL work together to prevent your shin from moving forward in relation to your thigh. Ideally, the hamstrings should absorb force produced during running, jumping and other athletic movements, but if your hamstrings are weak or dysfunctional, the ACL will have to pick up the slack. If your hamstrings are not working properly your risk of ACL-injury increases dramatically.

In addition to supporting the ACL, the hamstrings also take load of the front portion of the knee by preventing too much forward movement of the shinbone. This helps to avoid overload of the tissues on the front of the knee and thereby lowers your risk of developing overuse injuries in those regions.

The hamstrings play an important role in sports. With strong hamstrings, you will run faster, jump higher, and you're less likely to get injured.

Good ankle mobility

The ankles are part of our natural shock absorbers. The play a crucial role in determining the force distribution of impact forces through our legs, since they are the first major joint group between our body and the ground. Restrictions of ankle mobility will always come at the cost of preventing them from doing their job properly, which is one reason why ankle mobility needs to be trained.

Additionally, if we miss range of motion at the ankle, the body will increase the range of motion at the neighboring joint: the knee! This puts undue stress on the knee and increases your chances of developing knee pain.

Many things come into play when dealing with ankle range of motion. For example wearing any type of elevated heel will gradually decrease your ankle range of motion. The more elevated your heels, the worse your ankle mobility, the more likely you are to develop knee pain. Furthermore, the muscles that control movement around the ankle have become severely deconditioned due to restrictive footwear and lack of exercise diversity (*e.g.*, when was the last time you had to pull your toes up towards your knees?).

With the Total Knee Health program, you will restore full function to your ankles and have some fun in the process.

Good hip mobility

The muscles at the hip have a significant influence on knee position and controlled knee movement. Unfortunately, many of us have to deal with extended periods of sitting throughout the day and as result, our hip muscles are out of balance. In the majority of cases the hip flexors, adductors and hip internal rotators are tight, making it harder to resist excessive internal rotation, adduction, and forward translation of the tibia. This means you're more likely to end up with your knee collapsing inward and your shinbone travelling too far forward.

To get the most out of our gluteal and hamstring training, we also have to improve hip mobility. Optimizing hip mobility is like removing the handbrake, as tight hips slow you down in sports.

High skill at single-leg exercises

In daily life as well as in sports you frequently use only one leg at a time. In fact, our basic skills of locomotion, walking and running, require us to lift one leg off the ground. How much skill we display at those activities largely depends on how skillful we are at single-leg exercises. This can be as simple as lifting one foot a few centimeters off the ground without changing the alignment in the rest of your body.

Maintaining good body alignment during single-leg exercises is very demanding. This kind of training will increase your body awareness significantly and it allows you to overload your legs without having to use additional weight. Since you're only using one leg you can fully concentrate on ingraining proper alignment and the carry-over to sports will be tremendous.

Another benefit of single-leg training is the training effect it has on the muscles around your ankles and in your feet. Your balance will improve noticeably and your chances of spraining an ankle will drop. This is because your body learns how to react to the forces on the ankle to maintain proper alignment. A benefit that is completely lost when training in cushioned shoes.

The Total Knee Health program will carefully guide you through a progression of single-leg exercises.

Excellent soft-tissue quality

The term soft-tissue describes all the tissues in the body that support its non-skeletal parts such as organs. Soft-tissue includes muscles, tendons, ligaments, fascia and even tissues such as skin. There are healthcare professionals who will work on all these tissues to improve your health, but at home, we can only safely work on muscles.

When certain layers or soft-tissue don't behave as they should you can end up with problems such as knee pain. In this particular case, there might be soft-tissue restrictions in the legs, hips or other parts of the body. These could be adhesions between muscles or with other tissue. Such restrictions lower your movement quality by decreasing range of motion at affected joints. It's like the rope of a pulley being stuck because of a knot or the individual ropes of the pulley having been tangled up. To be able to use the pulley properly again you will have to untangle the ropes and remove the knot. In the case of soft-tissue restrictions this means manual manipulation of soft-tissue (*e.g.*, via massage, or self-massage).

Later in this book you will learn how you can improve your soft-tissue quality at home without having to spend more than a couple of minutes every day.

Unbalanced movement habits

"Comfort zone" is usually used in relation to behavioral patterns, but there's also a movement comfort zone. As we grow older, there's a natural tendency towards working our strengths and neglecting our weaknesses. The runners run, swimmers swim, tennis players play tennis, etc. Unfortunately, unbalanced movement habits will also lead to muscular imbalances, which in turn can lead to pain.

Another reason why we don't have a lot of variety in our movement is the fact that we've shaped our environments for highest possible convenience. Everything is as flat as possible, stairs make it easy to get to a higher place without having to use your upper body at all (is climbing stairs really climbing?) and as if all that weren't enough we can also have us transported everywhere. On one hand we try to exert ourselves as little as possible during the day leading to a deconditioned body, on the other hand we expect our body to cope with very demanding situations in sports leading to overuse injuries and pain.

Have you ever seen a cat stretch and warm up for 10 minutes before running after a mouse? Does a gazelle warm up before being chased by a cheetah? The cheetah goes from 0 to 60 mph (ca. 100 km/h) in about 3 seconds, so there's not a lot of time to warm up it seems. The reason why animals have to neither warm up nor stretch is that they move all day in a wide variety of ways. Their bodies are primed for high performance during all of their waking hours. Everything else would equal extinction sooner, rather than later.

Our goal should be to balance our movements. For every vertical push you do, you should add some vertical pulling into your program. The same goes for horizontal pressing and pulling, but also for upright walking and locomotion in other stances. Think crouched walking, crawling on your stomach, walking on all fours with your back or your stomach to the ground etc. This variety will expose weaknesses, prepare you for the unlikely eventualities of your sport (or daily life) and make you more injury-proof. It's also a simple and effective workout.

Depending on the condition your knees are in you will have to approach this state of balance slowly, as too radical changes always increase your risk for injury. For this reason, we will progress very carefully towards reclaiming the state of movement versatility.

High movement quality

To be healthy and pain-free we need a certain degree of variety in our movement habits, but we also need a high movement quality when we move. The better your body alignment is, the more optimal the force distribution throughout your body will be. If your alignment is bad you will overload certain tissues (muscles, tendons, ligaments, etc.), while not placing enough load to stimulate adaptation on certain other tissues. Low movement quality could be knees that are collapsing inward when you're landing from a jump or the inability to absorb force efficiently (*e.g.*, making a lot of noise when landing from a jump or running).

To improve your movement quality you first have to become of aware of it. Next, you could use objective measures such as video recordings to judge it. With increased awareness, you can also judge the quality of your movement by how graceful it feels.

This may sound complicated, but all it really means is practicing movement in a variety of ways and always paying attention to maintaining high movement quality. Of course, this precludes going jogging with your MP3-player and having your mind wander from your running to what's for dinner. Movement practice always has to be mindful, with as few distractions as possible.

Are you competing or training?

At the "Fundamentals of Human Movement" seminar in Cologne Steve Maxwell posed a very interesting question about training: "How can you compete in training?" Since training is merely a means to an end, it makes absolutely no sense to compete in training. It doesn't matter who can do the most pushups, because as soon as you start competing in pushups technique will go right out of the window. As technique goes, your risk of injury increases. You are now working to achieve the opposite of what you originally were training for (*e.g.*, to get stronger and healthier).

As shaving is a means to get rid of hair, the pushup is a way to increase upper body strength. Nobody would think about competing in shaving to see who shaves the fastest, yet in training competition is common practice. This is something to keep in mind the next time you are challenged to a competition in training.

Reasonable increase in training loads

Different parts of the human body take a different time to adapt to the training stimulus. The central nervous system adapts quickly for example, but the adaptation of ligaments, tendons and bones takes much longer. Whenever you overtax your body, the weakest link in the chain will take damage. For example, maybe your muscles are strong enough to play 90 minutes of basketball, but your tendons aren't. In that case you will cause tissue damage to the affected tendons and while this is not noticeable the first couple of times it happens, you will start feeling discomfort at some point. At that point the physical damage to the tendon has already been done.

What this means is that you should always let your mind overrule your ego when it comes to sports. Don't play 90 minutes of basketball when you know you can only handle 45. Don't run a 10K when all you ever did was a 5K. As long as you increase your training loads reasonably, you won't hurt yourself. Aim for a maximum increase of 10% per week. For example, keeping your sets, reps and tempo constant you could increase the weight by 10%. Coming back to the basketball example, you could choose to play 45 minutes this week and 50 minutes next week.

Are you working out or are you practicing movement?

The mindset that has helped me most with avoiding the mentality of trying to achieve more by doing too much too soon was to think about training as movement practice, as opposed to "working out". Once you place your emphasis more on technique you will automatically stop once technique degrades past a certain point and as you adapt this habit, you will avoid being injured. The lower risk of injury results from the increased movement quality. It's also worth remembering that the more fatigued you get, the lower your movement quality will be and the more you run the risk of injury.

How Stretching Actually Works

This excerpt explains why certain muscles, like the ones in your hip, become stiff over time and why moving a joint through its full range of motion is important if you don't want to lose mobility. Total Knee Health, chapter 4 excerpt:

The common misconception about stretching is that it works by physically lengthening the involved tissues. There is some truth to that, as the length of the involved tissues really increases during stretching, but soon after the activity stops it will return to its previous length. How long this takes depends on hard and long you were stretching, but your muscles will generally be back to their regular length within 10 minutes.

The mechanism by which your flexibility is actually determined is based on how muscles work. Muscles are built of tiny threads of protein that slide against each other to cause contractions. This process is largely controlled by your central nervous system (NB: the unbelievable amount of computing power it requires to coordinate the actions of over 600 muscles in our bodies based on complex sensory input to create sophisticated movement is astounding to say the least).

At birth, we all start with no knowledge on how to control our movements. The central nervous system first has to learn how to use each muscle and how to coordinate muscle actions to create controlled movement. As this learning process takes place, more and more information on how to create movement is stored. The brain also "remembers" which muscle length ranges are preferably used. The activities a child performs will leave a strong imprint on their athletic potential.

On the flipside, inactivity as a child will make it significantly harder for that person to learn new movements in the future. When it comes to actual motor control, a good example for this is throwing a ball. Some children never do a lot of throwing. As adults, they will not be able to throw objects and it will be difficult for them learn. Children that do a lot of throwing only throw with one side, so the other side will be weak and uncoordinated.

The connection to stretching is based on the ranges of preferred length that our central nervous system stores. When a person is conscious, their CNS continuously monitors length and movement of muscles. If the CNS detects a muscle that is extending beyond what has been stored as the standard length, it will automatically create tension in the muscle to protect you from injury. This is illustrated by the unlimited flexibility that unconscious people exhibit. Their limbs can be moved without restriction from the muscles as long as the person is unconscious, but when they wake up their nervous system will seize control over the muscles yet again and the previous feats of flexibility will be impossible.

The way stretching actually works is by retraining the nervous system and "proving" to it, repeatedly, that a certain muscle length is safe. There are several different ways to do this and each has different advantages. Later you will learn some methods with which you can efficiently increase your own flexibility, but remember that every move you make stands against millions of movements you've made in your past. Based on how active you have been in your life, your range of flexibility will be different. It's a question of persistence in "retraining" the central nervous system, which means regular practice is essential.

You've Fixed Your Jumper's Knee. Now What?

To stay up to date, join my free email course on the most common causes for knee pain. It's an excellent companion for this book and it will help you stay on track with healing your jumper's knee. Additionally, there is always some new and exciting research around the corner when it comes to patellar tendonitis. If you're signed on the email course, you'll be the first to know about new treatment approaches for patellar tendonitis.

You can find the course on your online resources page:

http://www.fix-knee-pain.com/jumpers-knee-book-guide

Your Blueprint to Keeping Your Knees Healthy for Life

In this book, you've discovered science-based techniques and exercises that will help you heal your patellar tendonitis and prevent it from returning in the future. You now know more about jumper's knee than doctors learn in medical school. If history is of any indication, it will take a few more decades until this knowledge becomes part of the curriculum, unless a miracle happens.

There has always been a gap between what science knows and what people in the field actually believe and do, regardless of whether it's in the medical profession, business, pedagogy, or other areas.

Is the earth flat or round?

Is it possible to build a flying machine?

Is it ok to hit children that misbehave or are there better ways to teach them?

Certain ideas are ahead of their time and only a few individuals benefit by applying them, while everyone else is shaking their head in disbelief, foregoing advantages they literally can't imagine. Using this knowledge "from the future" will give you an advantage in all areas of life and getting this knowledge often is as easy as buying a book.

For knee health, I can offer you more knowledge "from the future" if you're interested. In my book Total Knee Health, you will learn about other hidden causes for knee pain and you'll be given the tools to keep your knees healthy for life. Here are some of its topics:

- How dietary choices can destroy your cartilage and cause arthritis
- How proper breathing helps relax your muscles and keeps your joints healthy (and how to do it)
- Lifestyle cheats you can use to improve your recovery and boost your performance
- Which kinds of shoes will ruin your children's feet for life and cause collapsed arches and knee pain
- A brutally efficient (but safe!) exercise the Soviet special forces use to strengthen their legs, knees, and spirit (plus countless other knee health exercises)
- … and more

Total Knee Health captures everything I've learned about knees by training with world-class coaches, reading research, and experimenting on myself, over the last three years. The feedback I've gotten from readers has been overwhelming and I was even invited to share this knowledge with the German National Volleyball team. Here are just two reader emails I've gotten about Total Knee Health:

> "Martin Koban, I downloaded your book, read it, and have been doing the exercises suggested and all I can say is 'GREAT JOB'. I am 61 years old and I have had 3 surgeries on my knees as a result of playing American football in high school and college. I also coach football and basketball and we are having our team use these exercises. Once again thank you for your outstanding research and making it available to us."
> – George Whary

"Your ebook is incredible! You should have titled your book, 'Everything you need to know about your knee but your doctor didn't tell you OR didn't know!' You are really providing people like me with information they can't get anywhere else-this could change my life! It gives me some hope that maybe my knee can get better!"
– Susan Pech

If you want to speed up your healing and keep your knees healthy for life by using more knowledge "from the future," you should definitely check out my book Total Knee Health.

It's only available through my website:

http://www.total-knee-health.com/

(Redirects to fix-knee-pain.com)

Acknowledgements

I didn't come up with most of the ideas in this book and the long list of references stands testimony to that. In particular, I would like to thank the following people for their (indirect) contribution to this book. This book wouldn't have been possible without your help and inspiration. Thank you!

Steve Maxwell, http://www.maxwellsc.com/

Dr. Kelly Starrett, http://www.mobilitywod.com/

Dr. Perry Nickelston, http://www.painlasercenter.com/

Mike Robertson, http://robertsontrainingsystems.com/

Vladimir Vasiliev, http://www.russianmartialart.com/

Erwan LeCorre, http://www.movnat.com/

Ido Portal, http://www.idoportal.com/

Tim Ferriss, http://www.fourhourworkweek.com/blog/

Thank you Jennifer Chase, for being an awesome editor and helping me improve this book.

Lastly, I want to thank all researchers quoted in this book. Your research provided the foundation for helping countless athletes to recover from jumper's knee and as such, I would like to express my highest gratitude for your continued efforts in finding better ways to treat injuries.

(Please note: At the time of this writing, none of the individuals mentioned here endorse this book.)

Thank you

Before you go, I'd like to say "thank you" for purchasing this book and reading it all the way to the end.

Now, I'd like to ask you for a **small** favor. Could you please take a minute and leave a review for this book on Amazon:

http://www.fix-knee-pain.com/jumpers-knee-book
(Forwards to Amazon)

Your feedback will help strangers from around the globe find the answers they need to fix their jumper's knee and will keep me motivated to dig up more tricks to beat this stubborn injury.

If you've loved the book, please let me know through a review on Amazon.

Thank You!

References

A Prospective Randomized Study Comparing the Therapeutic Effect of Tendoactive®, Eccentric Training, and a Combination of Both as a Treatment of Achilles Tendinopathy - ICH GCP - Clinical Trials Registry. Available online at http://ichgcp.net/clinical-trials-registry/research/index/NCT01691716, checked on 4/07/2013.

Tendonitis - Mobility - GymnasticBodies. Available online at https://www.gymnasticbodies.com/forum/topic/741-tendonitis/, checked on 3/07/2013.

Aiyegbusi, Ayoola I.; Olabiyi, Olaleye O.; Duru, Francis I. O.; Noronha, Cressie C.; Okanlawon, Abayomi O. (2011): A comparative study of the effects of bromelain and fresh pineapple juice on the early phase of healing in acute crush achilles tendon injury. In *J Med Food* 14 (4), pp. 348–352.

Alfredson, H.; Pietilä, T.; Jonsson, P.; Lorentzon, R. (1998): Heavy-load eccentric calf muscle training for the treatment of chronic Achilles tendinosis. In *Am J Sports Med* 26 (3), pp. 360–366.

Andres, Brett M.; Murrell, George A. C. (2008): Treatment of tendinopathy: what works, what does not, and what is on the horizon. In *Clin. Orthop. Relat. Res.* 466 (7), pp. 1539–1554.

Backman, Ludvig J.; Danielson, Patrik (2011): Low range of ankle dorsiflexion predisposes for patellar tendinopathy in junior elite basketball players: a 1-year prospective study. In *Am J Sports Med* 39 (12), pp. 2626–2633.

Bisseling, R. W.; Hof, A. L.; Bredeweg, S. W.; Zwerver, J.; Mulder, T. (2007): Relationship between landing strategy and patellar tendinopathy in volleyball. In *British Journal of Sports Medicine* 41 (7), pp. e8.

Bjørkkjaer, T.; Brunborg, L. A.; Arslan, G.; Lind, R. A.; Brun, J. G.; Valen, M. et al. (2004): Reduced joint pain after short-term duodenal administration of seal oil in patients with inflammatory bowel disease: comparison with soy oil. In *Scand. J. Gastroenterol.* 39 (11), pp. 1088–1094.

Buhrmann, Constanze; Mobasheri, Ali; Busch, Franziska; Aldinger, Constance; Stahlmann, Ralf; Montaseri, Azadeh; Shakibaei, Mehdi

(2011): Curcumin modulates nuclear factor kappaB (NF-kappaB)-mediated inflammation in human tenocytes in vitro: role of the phosphatidylinositol 3-kinase/Akt pathway. In *J. Biol. Chem.* 286 (32), pp. 28556–28566.

Cannell, L. J. (2001): A randomised clinical trial of the efficacy of drop squats or leg extension/leg curl exercises to treat clinically diagnosed jumper's knee in athletes: pilot study. In *British Journal of Sports Medicine* 35 (1), pp. 60–64.

Cardone, Dennis A.: Is Platelet-Rich Plasma an Effective Healing Therapy?: Scientific American. Available online at http://www.scientificamerican.com/article.cfm?id=platelet-rich-plasma-therapy-dennis-cardone-sports-medicine-injury&page=2, checked on 8/07/2013.

Carter, Jason R.; Schwartz, Christopher E.; Yang, Huan; Joyner, Michael J. (2013): Fish oil and neurovascular reactivity to mental stress in humans. In *Am. J. Physiol. Regul. Integr. Comp. Physiol.* 304 (7), pp. R523-30.

Caturla, Nuria; Funes, Lorena; Pérez-Fons, Laura; Micol, Vicente (2011): A randomized, double-blinded, placebo-controlled study of the effect of a combination of lemon verbena extract and fish oil omega-3 fatty acid on joint management. In *J Altern Complement Med* 17 (11), pp. 1051–1063.

Chester, Rachel; Costa, Mathew L.; Shepstone, Lee; Cooper, Adele; Donell, Simon T. (2008): Eccentric calf muscle training compared with therapeutic ultrasound for chronic Achilles tendon pain--a pilot study. In *Man Ther* 13 (6), pp. 484–491.

Cook, J. L. (2001): What is the most appropriate treatment for patellar tendinopathy? In *British Journal of Sports Medicine* 35 (5), pp. 291–294.

Cook, J. L.; Purdam, C. R. (2009): Is tendon pathology a continuum? A pathology model to explain the clinical presentation of load-induced tendinopathy. In *British Journal of Sports Medicine* 43 (6), pp. 409–416.

Cressey, Eric (2006): Truth About Leg Extensions. Available online at http://www.t-nation.com/free_online_article/sports_body_training_performance_repair/the_truth_about_leg_extensions, updated on 7/11/2006, checked on 18/06/2013.

Deal, C. L.; Moskowitz, R. W. (1999): Nutraceuticals as therapeutic agents in osteoarthritis. The role of glucosamine, chondroitin sulfate, and collagen hydrolysate. In *Rheum. Dis. Clin. North Am.* 25 (2), pp. 379–395.

Delarue, J.; Matzinger, O.; Binnert, C.; Schneiter, P.; Chioléro, R.; Tappy, L. (2003): Fish oil prevents the adrenal activation elicited by mental stress in healthy men. In *Diabetes Metab.* 29 (3), pp. 289–295.

Fearon, A. M.; Cook, J. L.; Smith, P.; Scott, A. (2013): GENE EXPRESSION IN TENOCYTES SUGGESTS DEGNERATIVE TENDON TEARS ATTEMPT TO HEAL. In *British Journal of Sports Medicine* 47 (9), pp. e2.

Frohm, A.; Saartok, T.; Halvorsen, K.; Renstrom, P. (2007): Eccentric treatment for patellar tendinopathy: a prospective randomised short-term pilot study of two rehabilitation protocols. In *British Journal of Sports Medicine* 41 (7), pp. e7.

Furia, John P.; Rompe, Jan D.; Cacchio, Angelo; Del Buono, Angelo; Maffulli, Nicola (2013): A single application of low-energy radial extracorporeal shock wave therapy is effective for the management of chronic patellar tendinopathy. In *Knee Surg Sports Traumatol Arthrosc* 21 (2), pp. 346–350.

Gaida, J. E.; Cook, J. L.; Bass, S. L.; Austen, S.; Kiss, Z. S. (2004): Are unilateral and bilateral patellar tendinopathy distinguished by differences in anthropometry, body composition, or muscle strength in elite female basketball players? In *Br J Sports Med* 38 (5), pp. 581–585.

Garau, Giorgio; Rittweger, Joern; Mallarias, Peter; Longo, Umile Giuseppe; Maffulli, Nicola (2008): Traumatic patellar tendinopathy. In *Disabil Rehabil* 30 (20-22), pp. 1616–1620.

Goldberg, Robert J.; Katz, Joel (2007): A meta-analysis of the analgesic effects of omega-3 polyunsaturated fatty acid supplementation for inflammatory joint pain. In *Pain* 129 (1-2), pp. 210–223.

Grau, S.; Maiwald, C.; Krauss, I.; Axmann, D.; Janssen, P.; Horstmann, T. (2008): What are causes and treatment strategies for patellar-tendinopathy in female runners? In *J Biomech* 41 (9), pp. 2042–2046.

Grosso, Giuseppe; Bei, Roberto; Mistretta, Antonio; Marventano, Stefano; Calabrese, Giorgio; Masuelli, Laura et al. (2013): Effects of

Vitamin C on health: a review of evidence. In *Front. Biosci.* 18, pp. 1017–1029.

Guebre-Egziabher, Fitsum; Debard, Cyril; Drai, Jocelyne; Denis, Laure; Pesenti, Sandra; Bienvenu, Jacques et al. (2013): Differential dose effect of fish oil on inflammation and adipose tissue gene expression in chronic kidney disease patients. In *Nutrition* 29 (5), pp. 730–736.

Hägglund, Martin; Zwerver, Johannes; Ekstrand, Jan (2011): Epidemiology of patellar tendinopathy in elite male soccer players. In *Am J Sports Med* 39 (9), pp. 1906–1911.

Hall, Micheal P.; Ward, James P.; Cardone, Dennis A. (2013): Platelet Rich Placebo? Evidence for Platelet Rich Plasma in the Treatment of Tendinopathy and Augmentation of Tendon Repair. In *Bulletin of the Hospital for Joint Diseases* 71.

Hellhammer, Juliane; Hero, Torsten; Franz, Nadin; Contreras, Carina; Schubert, Melanie (2012): Omega-3 fatty acids administered in phosphatidylserine improved certain aspects of high chronic stress in men. In *Nutr Res* 32 (4), pp. 241–250.

Huisman, E.; Thornton, G.; Roberts, C.; Scott, A. (2013): IDENTIFICATION OF BIOMARKERS FOR EARLY TENDON DEGENERATION USING AN IN-VIVO RABBIT MODEL. In *British Journal of Sports Medicine* 47 (9), pp. e2.

Ireland, Mary Lloyd; Willson, John D.; Ballantyne, Bryon T.; Davis, Irene McClay (2003): Hip strength in females with and without patellofemoral pain. In *J Orthop Sports Phys Ther* 33 (11), pp. 671–676.

Jainu, Mallika; Devi, C.S Shyamala (2005): In Vitro. and In Vivo. Evaluation of Free-Radical Scavenging Potential of Cissus quadrangularis. In *Pharmaceutical Biology* 43 (9), pp. 773–779.

Jonsson, P. (2005): Superior results with eccentric compared to concentric quadriceps training in patients with jumper's knee: a prospective randomised study. In *British Journal of Sports Medicine* 39 (11), pp. 847–850.

Kannus, P. (2000): Structure of the tendon connective tissue. In *Scand J Med Sci Sports* 10 (6), pp. 312–320.

Kannus, P.; Józsa, L. (1991): Histopathological changes preceding spontaneous rupture of a tendon. A controlled study of 891 patients. In *J Bone Joint Surg Am* 73 (10), pp. 1507–1525.

Kettunen, Jyrki A.; Kvist, Martti; Alanen, Erkki; Kujala, Urho M. (2002): Long-term prognosis for jumper's knee in male athletes. A prospective follow-up study. In *Am J Sports Med* 30 (5), pp. 689–692.

Khan, K. M.; Maffulli, N.; Coleman, B. D.; Cook, J. L.; Taunton, J. E. (1998): Patellar tendinopathy: some aspects of basic science and clinical management. In *Br J Sports Med* 32 (4), pp. 346–355.

Kipp, D. E.; McElvain, M.; Kimmel, D. B.; Akhter, M. P.; Robinson, R. G.; Lukert, B. P. (1996): Scurvy results in decreased collagen synthesis and bone density in the guinea pig animal model. In *Bone* 18 (3), pp. 281–288.

Kongsgaard, M.; Kovanen, V.; Aagaard, P.; Doessing, S.; Hansen, P.; Laursen, A. H. et al. (2009): Corticosteroid injections, eccentric decline squat training and heavy slow resistance training in patellar tendinopathy. In *Scand J Med Sci Sports* 19 (6), pp. 790–802.

Kongsgaard, Mads; Qvortrup, Klaus; Larsen, Jytte; Aagaard, Per; Doessing, Simon; Hansen, Philip et al. (2010): Fibril morphology and tendon mechanical properties in patellar tendinopathy: effects of heavy slow resistance training. In *Am J Sports Med* 38 (4), pp. 749–756.

Kubo, Keitaro; Ikebukuro, Toshihiro; Yata, Hideaki; Tsunoda, Naoya; Kanehisa, Hiroaki (2010): Time course of changes in muscle and tendon properties during strength training and detraining. In *J Strength Cond Res* 24 (2), pp. 322–331.

Larsson, Maria E. H.; Käll, Ingela; Nilsson-Helander, Katarina (2012): Treatment of patellar tendinopathy—a systematic review of randomized controlled trials. In *Knee Surg Sports Traumatol Arthrosc* 20 (8), pp. 1632–1646.

Lavagnino, Michael; Arnoczky, Steven P.; Elvin, Niell; Dodds, Julie (2008): Patellar tendon strain is increased at the site of the jumper's knee lesion during knee flexion and tendon loading: results and cadaveric testing of a computational model. In *Am J Sports Med* 36 (11), pp. 2110–2118.

Lewis, Jeremy S.; Sandford, Fiona M. (2009): Rotator Cuff Tendinopathy: Is There a Role for Polyunsaturated Fatty Acids and Antioxidants? In *Journal of Hand Therapy* 22 (1), pp. 49–56.

Lian, Oystein B.; Engebretsen, Lars; Bahr, Roald (2005): Prevalence of jumper's knee among elite athletes from different sports: a cross-sectional study. In *Am J Sports Med* 33 (4), pp. 561–567.

Lian, Øystein; Refsnes, Per-Egil; Engebretsen, Lars; Bahr, Roald (2003): Performance characteristics of volleyball players with patellar tendinopathy. In *Am J Sports Med* 31 (3), pp. 408–413.

Lippiello, Louis (2007): Collagen Synthesis in tenocytes, ligament cells and chondrocytes exposed to a combination of Glucosamine HCl and chondroitin sulfate. In *Evid Based Complement Alternat Med* 4 (2), pp. 219–224.

Magnusson, S. Peter; Langberg, Henning; Kjaer, Michael (2010): The pathogenesis of tendinopathy: balancing the response to loading. In *Nat Rev Rheumatol* 6 (5), pp. 262–268.

Maia Filho, Antonio Luiz Martins; Villaverde, Antonio Balbin; Munin, Egberto; Aimbire, Flávio; Albertini, Regiane (2010): Comparative study of the topical application of Aloe vera gel, therapeutic ultrasound and phonophoresis on the tissue repair in collagenase-induced rat tendinitis. In *Ultrasound Med Biol* 36 (10), pp. 1682–1690.

Malliaras, Peter; Cook, Jillianne L.; Kent, Peter (2006): Reduced ankle dorsiflexion range may increase the risk of patellar tendon injury among volleyball players. In *J Sci Med Sport* 9 (4), pp. 304–309.

Manias, P.; Stasinopoulos, D. (2006): A controlled clinical pilot trial to study the effectiveness of ice as a supplement to the exercise programme for the management of lateral elbow tendinopathy. In *Br J Sports Med* 40 (1), pp. 81–85.

Mann, Kerry J.; Edwards, Suzi; Drinkwater, Eric J.; Bird, Stephen P. (2013): A lower limb assessment tool for athletes at risk of developing patellar tendinopathy. In *Med Sci Sports Exerc* 45 (3), pp. 527–533.

Omeroğlu, Suna; Peker, Tuncay; Türközkan, Nurten; Omeroğlu, Hakan (2009): High-dose vitamin C supplementation accelerates the Achilles tendon healing in healthy rats. In *Arch Orthop Trauma Surg* 129 (2), pp. 281–286.

Ozer, Hamza; Taşkesen, Anıl; Kul, Oğuz; Selek, Hakan Y.; Turanlı, Sacit; Köse, Kenan (2011): Glukozamin kondroitin sülfatın onarılmış tenotomize sıçan Aşil tendonları üzerine etkisi. In *Eklem Hastalik Cerrahisi* 22 (2), pp. 100–106.

Poliquin, Charles: Why Fish Oils Are The Most Important Supplement - Charles Poliquin. Available online at http://www.charlespoliquin.com/Blog/tabid/130/EntryId/118/Why-Fish-Oils-Are-The-Most-Important-Supplement.aspx, checked on 13/05/2013.

Poliquin, Charles (2006): T NATION | Question of Strength: Vol 35. Available online at http://www.t-nation.com/free_online_article/sports_body_training_performance/question_of_strength_december_06, updated on 23/12/2006, checked on 4/07/2013.

Portal, Ido: The Importance of Supplementation for Athletes - Nutrition - GymnasticBodies. Available online at https://www.gymnasticbodies.com/forum/topic/3190-the-importance-of-supplementation-for-athletes/, checked on 4/07/2013.

Powers, Christopher M. (2010): The influence of abnormal hip mechanics on knee injury: a biomechanical perspective. In *J Orthop Sports Phys Ther* 40 (2), pp. 42–51.

Purdam, C. R. (2004): A pilot study of the eccentric decline squat in the management of painful chronic patellar tendinopathy. In *British Journal of Sports Medicine* 38 (4), pp. 395–397.

Purdam, Craig R.; Cook, Jill L.; Hopper, Diana M.; Khan, Karim M.; VIS tendon study group (2003): Discriminative ability of functional loading tests for adolescent jumper's knee. In *Physical Therapy in Sport* 4 (1), pp. 3–9.

Rees, J. D.; Stride, M.; Scott, A. (2013): TENDONS: TIME TO REVISIT INFLAMMATION? In *British Journal of Sports Medicine* 47 (9), pp. e2.

Reeves, N. D.; Maganaris, C. N.; Narici, M. V. (2003): Effect of strength training on human patella tendon mechanical properties of older individuals. In *J. Physiol. (Lond.)* 548 (Pt 3), pp. 971–981.

Rompe, J. D.; Nafe, B.; Furia, J. P.; Maffulli, N. (2006): Eccentric Loading, Shock-Wave Treatment, or a Wait-and-See Policy for

Tendinopathy of the Main Body of Tendo Achillis: A Randomized
Controlled Trial. In *The American Journal of Sports Medicine* 35 (3), pp.
374–383.

Rompe, Jan D. (2008): Eccentric Loading Compared with Shock Wave
Treatment for Chronic Insertional Achilles TendinopathyA
Randomized, Controlled Trial. In *J Bone Joint Surg Am* 90 (1), p. 52.

Rompe, Jan D.; Maffulli, Nicola (2007): Repetitive shock wave therapy
for lateral elbow tendinopathy (tennis elbow): a systematic and
qualitative analysis. In *Br. Med. Bull.* 83, pp. 355–378.

Rowe, Victoria; Hemmings, Stephanie; Barton, Christian; Malliaras,
Peter; Maffulli, Nicola; Morrissey, Dylan (2012): Conservative
management of midportion Achilles tendinopathy: a mixed methods
study, integrating systematic review and clinical reasoning. In *Sports Med*
42 (11), pp. 941–967.

Russell, J. E.; Manske, P. R. (1991): Ascorbic acid requirement for
optimal flexor tendon repair in vitro. In *J. Orthop. Res.* 9 (5), pp. 714–
719.

Rutland, Marsha; O'Connell, Dennis; Brismée, Jean-Michel; Sizer, Phil;
Apte, Gail; O'Connell, Janelle (2010): Evidence-supported
rehabilitation of patellar tendinopathy. In *N Am J Sports Phys Ther* 5 (3),
pp. 166–178.

Scorei, Romulus; Mitrut, Paul; Petrisor, Iulian; Scorei, Iulia (2011): A
double-blind, placebo-controlled pilot study to evaluate the effect of
calcium fructoborate on systemic inflammation and dyslipidemia
markers for middle-aged people with primary osteoarthritis. In *Biol
Trace Elem Res* 144 (1-3), pp. 253–263.

Shakibaei, M.; Buhrmann, C.; Mobasheri, A. (2011): Anti-inflammatory
and anti-catabolic effects of TENDOACTIVE® on human tenocytes
in vitro. In *Histol. Histopathol.* 26 (9), pp. 1173–1185.

Sharma, Pankaj; Maffulli, Nicola (2008): Tendinopathy and tendon
injury: The future. In *Disabil Rehabil* 30 (20-22), pp. 1733–1745.

Smith, M. M.; Ravi, V.; Dart, A. J.; Sonnabend, D. H.; Little, C. B.
(2013): FACTORS AFFECTING TENDINOPATHOGENESIS. In
British Journal of Sports Medicine 47 (9), pp. e2.

Smith, R. K. W. (2013): STEM CELL THERAPY FOR
TENDINOPATHY: LESSONS FROM A LARGE ANIMAL
MODEL. In *British Journal of Sports Medicine* 47 (9), pp. e2.

Sofi, Francesco; Giorgi, Gianluca; Cesari, Francesca; Gori, Anna Maria;
Mannini, Lucia; Parisi, Giuliana et al. (2013): The atherosclerotic risk
profile is affected differently by fish flesh with a similar EPA and DHA
content but different n-6/n-3 ratio. In *Asia Pac J Clin Nutr* 22 (1), pp.
32–40.

Sommer, Christopher: Achilles tendonitis - CrossFit Discussion Board.
Available online at
http://board.crossfit.com/showthread.php?t=14890, checked on
3/07/2013.

Stanish, W. D.; Rubinovich, R. M.; Curwin, S. (1986): Eccentric
exercise in chronic tendinitis. In *Clin. Orthop. Relat. Res.* (208), pp. 65–
68.

Starkey, Jonathan: LiteCure Lasers Gaining Believers as Physical
Therapy Aid. Available online at http://www.delawarebio.org/litecure-
lasers-gaining-believers-as-physical-therapy-aid, checked on 7/07/2013.

Starrett, Kelly; Cordoza, Glen (2013): Becoming a Supple Leopard. The
Ultimate Guide to Resolving Pain, Preventing Injury, and Optimizing
Athletic Performance: Tuttle Publishing.

Stasinopoulos, Dimitrios; Stasinopoulos, Ioannis (2004): Comparison
of effects of exercise programme, pulsed ultrasound and transverse
friction in the treatment of chronic patellar tendinopathy. In *Clin
Rehabil* 18 (4), pp. 347–352.

Stohs, Sidney J.; Ray, Sidhartha D. (2012): A review and evaluation of
the efficacy and safety of Cissus quadrangularis extracts. In *Phytother
Res.*

Sussmilch-Leitch, Samuel P.; Collins, Natalie J.; Bialocerkowski,
Andrea E.; Warden, Stuart J.; Crossley, Kay M. (2012): Physical
therapies for Achilles tendinopathy: systematic review and meta-
analysis. In *J Foot Ankle Res* 5 (1), p. 15.

Tan, Suan Cheng; Chan, Otto (2008): Achilles and patellar
tendinopathy: Current understanding of pathophysiology and
management. In *Disabil Rehabil* 30 (20-22), pp. 1608–1615.

Tasto, James P.; Cummings, Jeffrey; Medlock, Virgil; Harwood, Frederick; Hardesty, Renee; Amiel, David (2003): The tendon treatment center: new horizons in the treatment of tendinosis. In *Arthroscopy: The Journal of Arthroscopic & Related Surgery* 19 (10), pp. 213–223.

Tiemessen, Ivo J. H.; Kuijer, P. Paul F. M.; Hulshof, Carel T. J.; Frings-Dresen, Monique H. W. (2009): Risk factors for developing jumper's knee in sport and occupation: a review. In *BMC Res Notes* 2, p. 127.

Tsai, Wen-Chung; Tang, Sf-T; Liang, Fang-Chen (2011): Effect of therapeutic ultrasound on tendons. In *Am J Phys Med Rehabil* 90 (12), pp. 1068–1073.

van Usen, Carla; Pumberger, Barbara (2007): Effectiveness of Eccentric Exercises in the Management of Chronic Achilles Tendinosis. In *The Internet Journal of Allied Health Sciences and Practice* 5 (2). Available online at http://ijahsp.nova.edu/articles/vol5num2/van_Usen.pdf.

Vangsness, C. Thomas; Spiker, William; Erickson, Juliana (2009): A review of evidence-based medicine for glucosamine and chondroitin sulfate use in knee osteoarthritis. In *Arthroscopy* 25 (1), pp. 86–94.

Vicenzino, B. (2013): THE CHALLENGE OF TENDON PAIN. In *British Journal of Sports Medicine* 47 (9), pp. e2.

Visnes, H.; Aandahl, H.; Bahr, R. (2013): JUMPING ABILITY AND CHANGE OF JUMPING ABILITY AS RISK FACTORS FOR DEVELOPING JUMPER'S KNEE. In *British Journal of Sports Medicine* 47 (9), pp. e2.

Visnes, Håvard; Bahr, Roald (2007): The evolution of eccentric training as treatment for patellar tendinopathy (jumper's knee): a critical review of exercise programmes. In *Br J Sports Med* 41 (4), pp. 217–223.

Visnes, Håvard; Hoksrud, Aasne; Cook, Jill; Bahr, Roald (2005): No effect of eccentric training on jumper's knee in volleyball players during the competitive season: a randomized clinical trial. In *Clin J Sport Med* 15 (4), pp. 227–234.

Warden, S. J.; Metcalf, B. R.; Kiss, Z. S.; Cook, J. L.; Purdam, C. R.; Bennell, K. L.; Crossley, K. M. (2008): Low-intensity pulsed ultrasound for chronic patellar tendinopathy: a randomized, double-blind, placebo-controlled trial. In *Rheumatology (Oxford)* 47 (4), pp. 467–471.

Wijesekera, Nevin T.; Chew, Ne Siang; Lee, Justin C.; Mitchell, Adam W.; Calder, James D.; Healy, Jeremiah C. (2010): Ultrasound-guided treatments for chronic Achilles tendinopathy: an update and current status. In *Skeletal Radiol.* 39 (5), pp. 425–434.

Wilson, John J.; Best, Thomas M. (2005): Common overuse tendon problems: A review and recommendations for treatment. In *Am Fam Physician* 72 (5), pp. 811–818.

Witvrouw, E.; Bellemans, J.; Lysens, R.; Danneels, L.; Cambier, D. (2001): Intrinsic risk factors for the development of patellar tendinitis in an athletic population. A two-year prospective study. In *Am J Sports Med* 29 (2), pp. 190–195.

Yamamoto, E.; Hayashi, K.; Yamamoto, N. (1999): Mechanical properties of collagen fascicles from stress-shielded patellar tendons in the rabbit. In *Clin Biomech (Bristol, Avon)* 14 (6), pp. 418–425.

Young, M. A. (2005): Eccentric decline squat protocol offers superior results at 12 months compared with traditional eccentric protocol for patellar tendinopathy in volleyball players. In *British Journal of Sports Medicine* 39 (2), pp. 102–105.

Index

Did you find this book useful? Please let me know by writing a review on Amazon:

http://www.fix-knee-pain.com/jumpers-knee-book
(Forwards to Amazon)

Thank You!